Progress in Orthopaedic Surgery

Vol. 5

Segmental Idiopathic Necrosis of the Femoral Head

Edited by U.H. Weil

Contributors
G. Buchhorn, Gottingen · P. Ficat, Toulouse
Y. Gérard, Rheims · Y. Hori, Kashihara, Nara
D.S. Hungerford, Baltimore · R. Kotz, Vienna
F.J. Wagenhäuser, Zurich · H. Wagner, Nuremberg/
Rummelsberg · H.G. Willert, Gottingen
G. Zeiler, Nuremberg/Rummelsberg
L. Zichner, Frankfurt on Main

With 68 Figures and 30 Tables

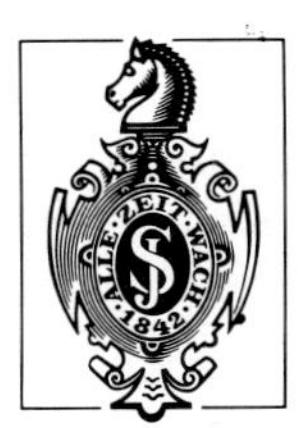

Springer-Verlag
Berlin Heidelberg New York 1981

Editor: U.H. Weil, M.D.
60 Temple Street, New Haven, Connecticut 06510 USA

ISBN 3-540-10718-5 Springer-Verlag Berlin Heidelberg New York
ISBN 0-387-10718-5 Springer-Verlag New York Heidelberg Berlin

Library of Congress Cataloging in Publication Data
Main entry under title:
Segmental idiopathic necrosis of the femoral head.
(Progress in orthopaedic surgery ; v. 5)
Includes index.
Contents: The question of posture / F.J. Wagenhäuser --
Early diagnosis of osteonecrosis by functional bone
investigation / P. Ficat -- Early diagnosis and treat-
ment of ischemic necrosis of the femoral head / D.S.
Hungerford -- [etc.]
1. Femur--Epiphysis--Surgery--Addresses, essays,
lectures. 2. Idiopathic femoral necrosis--Surgery--
Addresses, essays, lectures. I. Weil, U. H. (Ulrich
Henry) II. Buchhorn, G. III. Series. [DNLM:
1. Femur head necrosis. W1 PR677B v. 5 / WE 865 S454]
RD560.S43 1981 617'.582 81-16663
ISBN 0-387-10718-5 (U.S.) AACR2

Typesetting: Fotosatz Service Weihrauch, Würzburg
Printing and binding: Offsetdruckerei J. Beltz, Hemsbach
2125/3321-543210

Contents

Preface

Recent experience of the treatment of segmental idiopathic necrosis of the femoral head are discussed in this book by several experts. The discussed methods of treatment are practically unknown in the US orthopaedic literature. It describes alternate methods of treatment with regard to total joint replacement.

In Chapter 1 Dr. Wagenhäuser expresses his thoughts on posture and its affects on the human body. The following 7 chapters focus on diagnosis and treatment of idiopathic necrosis of the femoral head – an especially timely subject since the incidence of this disease, which primarily affects males during the most active period of their lives, seems to be increasing.

New Haven, Connecticut, August 1981 Ulrich H. Weil

The Question of Posture

F.J. Wagenhäuser

Every expert would agree with Taillard (1964) that posture is the most unsettled of all orthopaedic problems. Its onus of ambiguity no longer concerns orthopaedists alone, nor is it limited only to the fields of medical practice and research. It is, rather, a fundamental question spanning a wide range of sciences and occupations that deal with human existence and actions. Therefore fascination with this problem has steadily increased. Questions on human posture, its concepts and terminology, its normal forms and variations, the diagnosis of pathologic disorders, and their response to treatment concern many of today's anatomists, pathologists, physiologists, orthopaedists, rheumatologists, pediatricians, gerontologists, psychiatrists, psychosomatic therapists, physiologists, behavioral therapists, and epidemiologists. They are also the concern of school, military, occupational, preventive medicine, and space physicians, as well as parents, teachers, orthotherapists, physiotherapists, athletes, bioengineers, technical designers, and many others. Posture is obviously a human phenomenon that includes multiform anthropologic elements. Many of these aspects may be as enlightening as they are confusing. The problem of posture may be explained in many different ways depending on the point of view, visual angle, methodology, and the terminology employed. This can be very productive, but it can also lead to many misunderstandings.

The following necessarily incomplete explanations are limited to a few almost exclusively medical somatoclinical aspects of the problem. Hopefully they will shed some light on medical thinking concerning some fundamental principles of the question of posture.

Posture as a Problem of Evolution

Man's special nature is a direct cause of the problem of human posture. We agree with Schede (1969) and Steindler (1955) that human posture is a result and measure of the struggle between the pull of gravity and erect posture (Fig. 1). Man is the only organism which stands erect. Upright posture, together with more advanced development of the brain, particularly the cerebrum, and the development of speech and writing, is one of the most important recent acquisitions in the phylogenetic evolution of mankind. It seems that primates learned early to hold their trunk erect, but only man is capable of remaining upright for bipedal stance and movement. This specific bipedal form of upright posture freed man's upper extremities from the burden of locomotion and at the same time afforded him greater freedom to use his arms and particularly his hands for more refined

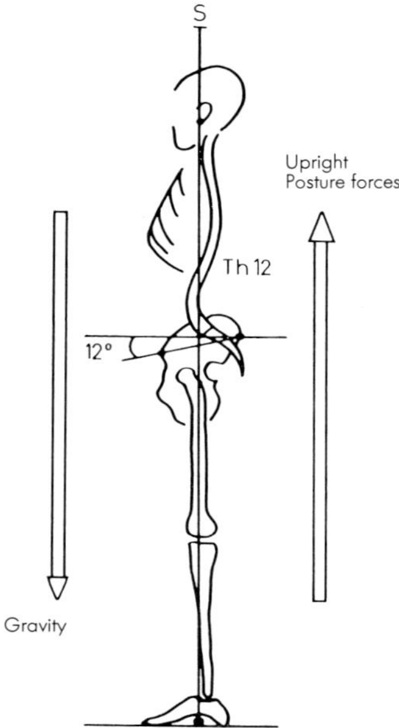

Fig. 1. Posture is an individual morphological and functional result of the struggle between the pull of gravity and the opposing forces of upright posture. S-line of gravity in normal habitual standing posture

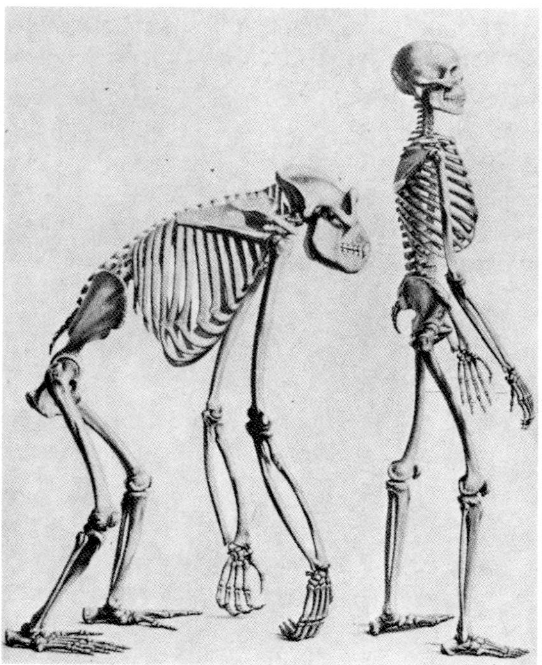

Fig. 2. The evolutionary step to the unique, erect posture of *Homo sapiens* is accompanied by specific new forms and structures in contrast to the primate

actions. Man could now not only *use* tools but also *make* them and even use them as weapons while walking or running. The unique static and dynamic properties of upright human posture were prerequisites for substantial development of the cranium and the enormous increase in the size of the cerebrum. Upright posture is therefore closely connected with the higher intellectual development and emancipation of *Homo sapiens*. Erect posture was also instrumental in widening the scope of man's eyesight to binocular, stereoscopic vision due to anterior placement of the eyes. Unlike quadrupeds and climbing anthropomorphous apes, man has a comprehensive optical, acoustic, and tactile awareness of this environment at his constant disposal.

It is obvious that erect posture, as an essential characteristic of mankind, is accompanied by specific new forms and structures. The human skeleton had to adjust to man's erect posture and movement (Fig. 2). Research into man's phylogenetic development led to the amazing discovery that human upright posture was not simply a result of a 90° rotation of the hip joint, but that it occurred mainly in the lumbosacral region as a result of a wedge-shaped transformation of the fifth lumbar and first sacral vertebrae (Lippert 1970). The sacrum is the immobile point around which the process of upright posture takes place. Human erect posture is the result of an angulation in the vertebral column, i.e., a result of upright displacement of the presacral section. The base of the sacrum lies at an acute angle to the anterior surface of the sacrum. This is unlike its position in quadrupeds, where the angle is almost perpendicular. Consequently, the promontorium, specific to man, is formed. The sharp angle between the sacrum and the lumbar section of the vertebral column is found only in man, and it is inherent (Benninghoff and Goerttler 1968). The pelvis and its fixed part, the sacrum, change position only slightly in comparison to quadrupeds in the total upright posture caused by the angle beneath the presacral cranial section of the spine.

The evolution of upright posture has produced a special form of the vertebral column. The double S-shape of the human vertebral column differs from the simple S-shape of the quadruped due to the supplementary lumbar lordosis. However, according to Lippert, it is not completely correct to consider this tendency to lumbar lordosis as essential for erect posture. Primarily, *functional* aspects seem to determine the double S-curve. From a functional point of view, it is evident that the S-shape of the vertebral column is the optimal configuration for demands of a dynamic nature (Leger 1959; Lippert 1970). Cervical and lumbar lordosis, together with thoracic kyphosis, work like interrelated springs. Massive deviations from these functionally adaptable curves are obviously mechanically unsuitable and result in increased and harmful functional strain. This is true for the excessively bent as well as for the excessively straight vertebral column.

Upright human posture obviously involves other specific anatomical forms which we will not discuss in detail but mention briefly in connection with man's total posture. Interestingly enough, the *position* of the pelvis plays only a minor part in man's upright posture. Conversely, its *shape*, which is unique to man, is connected with upright gait. The wide spread of the ilium is necessary for the origin of the gluteus maximus muscles, which are vital for upright human posture during standing or motion. It is well-known that this muscle is far less developed in anthropomorphous apes, which support themselves on their finger knuckles when standing or walking upright. The shape of the human thorax is also determined by upright posture and therefore differs quite considerably from that of quadrupeds. The respiratory mechanisms are closely linked to the movement of the spine. Conversely, all muscles associated with movement of the vertebral column also aid in respiration (Benninghoff and Goerttler 1968). During inspiration, there is constant concomitant innervation of the spinal column extensors as they adjust to the specific requirements of upright posture. These anatomical facts support clinical experience, which attaches considerable importance to breathing exercises in treatment of postural disorders.

The position of the scapula and rotation of the humerus should also be mentioned in connection with upright posture, since they are recently acquired specifically human attributes of the upper extremities. However, it is of interest that the construction of the human hand differs only slightly from that of the ape. Only its functional perfection and its superior powers of performance controlled by the central nervous system give the human hand its importance (Benninghoff and Goerttler 1968). Static and dynamic properties of the lower extremities have also undergone specific adjustments to upright posture. For example, the neck-shaft angle of the femur is unique to man; similarly, the torsions of the femoral shaft and the tibia, correlated to improve locomotion, are typically human features. However, the foot is the most important instrument which enables man to assume an upright stance and gait. Its special construction is not found in any other living organism. The human foot is not only required to *carry* the body but also to allow it to *move* by walking, running, or jumping. Its prehensile function was no longer needed and disappeared. The formation of the longitudinal arch is the most important process in the reconstruction of the foot to support human stance and gait. It is only due to the special construction of the longitudinal arch that man can assume his particular upright gait (Benninghoff and Goerttler).

The clinician should be reminded of the complex problem of posture by this short discussion of man's specific structural features, which are directly related to his unique, upright posture.

From a *phylogenetic* point of view, man obviously possesses many characteristic structural and functional attributes which are directly related to his upright posture. However, neither form nor function is totally provided for him at birth. Man's *ontogenetic development* is also unique since, unlike any other mammal, he has to make an "active conscious effort to learn and imitate" his particular posture for a long time after birth (Portmann 1969). This slow development of a normal total upright posture and of many basic morphological structures related to it is correlated with the evolvement of other physical, intellectual, and spiritual features as well as with his specific type of behavior. The characteristic features of upright human stance and gait are only partly inherent. Each individual must acquire and preserve most of them by constant learning, imitation, and eventually, "self-correction". As we have explained, the only inherent vital feature for the erect posture is the passively stabilized angle between the sacrum and the fifth lumbar vertebra in the region of the promontorium. Moreover, the vertebral column of a newborn child is straight and on the whole bent slightly backwards. Normal curves gradually evolve during the first 3 years of a child's life and by steady progression will become fixed during puberty. There is no doubt that the developing shape of the vertebral column is determined by a definite hereditary growth pattern. However, functional influences can modify this predetermined course of development (Lippert 1970).

Upright posture, granted to man through evolution, has afforded him such definite advantages that it must be considered to be an essential part or even a presupposition of man's special nature. Not without good reason did Haeckel consider erect posture to be such a specific human characteristic that he gave the name *Pithecanthropus erectus* to the "Primeval Ape-Man", which in his time was still a purely hypothetical creature. On the other hand, man has paid quite dearly for the unique advantage of upright posture and has obviously not yet mastered this stage of his evolution. His unique upright posture contributes not only to his supreme position in nature, but it also has a definite disorder potential whose significance we cannot yet fully perceive.

Posture as a Clinical Problem

The clinician must always realize that posture is the result of interaction among many kinds of factors. The term "posture" therefore represents an extremely complex collective concept, which must necessarily be divided into practical subconcepts. This division into individual elements is not only necessary for instruction purposes but also for diagnosis and treatment. However, this should never prevent one from considering posture in the final analysis as something total and self-contained. Despite all this, the most important clinical axiom should not be forgotten that "every posture represents a unique, individual, absolutely personal element of human nature". Everyone experiences a different result in the struggle between erect posture and the pull of gravity, making it an expression of his total physical and psychological personality. The multiplicity of individual postural forms is therefore not surprising, and it may easily be compared with the vast number of singularly human facial expression. In each particular case, posture is an individual, constantly changing solution to the situation of the moment, trying to provide the most stable body balance possible to counteract the pull of gravity. In practice, the clinician is obliged to work with different concepts of posture which we will discuss briefly. Justifiably, the spine is of central importance from the clinical view point. Nevertheless, it must be stressed that vertebral column posture is only one of the somatic elements of total posture. All other physical aspects of posture must also be considered in each assessment (Table 1). *Total human posture* is a result of the combination and interaction between *somatic and psychological aspects of posture.* Consequently, postural assessment requires not only isolated examination of the shape of the vertebral column, but also an assessment of the somatic and psychological aspects of the whole personality.

The particular individual body forms and forces by which man maintains erect balance against gravity constitute a *closed postural system* (Wagenhäuser 1972, 1977). This postural system is composed of structurally static and functionally dynamic elements coupled by reciprocal interaction. It creates an individualized postural pattern, which is always a personalized result of form and performance (Table 2). The particular shape of the vertebral column is of overriding importance among the elements of postural structure. The static, morphological, axial alignment of the vertebral column is provided by the particular shape and height of the vertebrae, by the position and direction of the vertebral arches with their articular, spinous, and transverse processes, and also by the height

Table 1. Total human posture

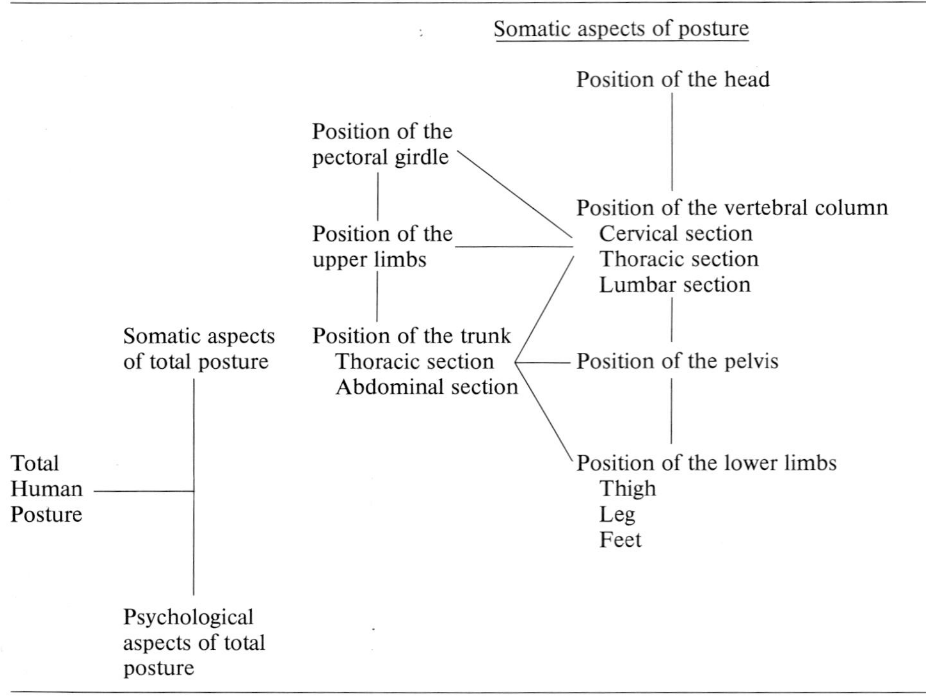

Table 2. Postural system

Structural static elements (Postural structure)	Reciprocal interaction	Functional dynamic elements (Postural performance)
Characteristic shape of the vertebral column		Musculature
		Coordination, postural
Shape of the thorax	Individual postural form	support by antigravity muscles
Shape of the pelvis	(personal postural pattern)	Tendons/Ligaments
Shape of the upper and lower limbs		Tautness, laxity
		Joint function
Joint structure		Range of motion
Somatomorphological constitution		Respiration
		Respiratory mechanism
		Central nervous system
		(Neuromuscular coordination)
		Pyramidal system
		(voluntary posture)
		Extrapyramidal system
		(involuntary posture)
		Sensory organs
		Eyes
		Inner ear (vestibular apparatus)
		Psychological constitution

and stability of the intervertebral discs. The characteristic structural form of the vertebral column, provided by the osseous spinal structures, intervertebral discs, and ligaments, is section easily identifiable as a single anatomical specimen. The preceding tried to explain that perfect upright posture presupposes not only a sound form of the vertebral column, but also quite specific forms of the thorax, pelvis, upper and lower extremities, and particularly of the feet. Any deviations in the characteristic shape of these structures will adversely affect and overburden the postural system. The so-called *antigravity muscles* are particularly important as a part of the functional dynamic elements of the postural system. They are the muscle groups which are used to hold and move the body in the most stable balance possible during upright posture and gait. These muscles do all the work of postural support. The greater the pull of gravity on postural balance, the harder they have to work. Muscle groups which stabilize the body's postural balance include not only the extensor muscles of the vertebral column, but also the neck muscles, pectoral girdle muscles, abdominal muscles, pelvic girdle muscles, and most importantly, the stabilizing muscle groups of the lower limbs and feet.

Efficient functioning of the dynamic postural system requires not only strong antigravity muscles, but also taut tendons and ligaments and sound neural control by the central nervous system. The central nervous system controls neuromuscular coordination and constantly adjusts to spontaneous demands by means of a complex reflex system. The most important sensory organs for assessment, control, and correction of posture are the eyes and the vestibular apparatus of the inner ear. Every clinician knows how seriously posture can be affected by a disorder of this neurologic control system. It has already been mentioned that the respiratory mechanism is actally part of the postural system. A sound postural system also requires functional efficiency, i.e., free joint motion. Restricted motion or even ankylosis, particularly of the hip, knee, or ankle joint, has a deleterious effect on posture.

In reviewing the whole postural system, one immediately comes to the conclusion that structural and functional disorders interact directly with each other. All static pathologic deviations cause a compensatory increase in neuromuscular functional exertion. With time, functional failure will also cause structural deterioration, and this creates a vicious circle. This is particularly true for the vertebral column. We have already mentioned that the normal S-shape of the vertebral column develops gradually during growth. Consequently, functional posture greatly influences static structural development. On the other hand, dynamic properties which determine form also have a definite modifying effect on the particular shape of the vertebral column during our entire life. Senile kyphosis and increased lumbar lordosis caused by weakened abdominal wall and gluteal muscles are classic examples of pathologic interaction between morbid postural shape and morbid postural performance. These close pathogenetic correlations are fundamentally important, not only for postural assessment but also particularly for orthotherapy. Conservative treatment of postural disorders is primarily based on correction and improvement of postural performance. It profits from the extremely important fact that posture is not something which is irreversibly fixed, but something which is continually changing. After all, every form of posture is an initial stage of movement that will result in a different posture.

Three basic terms are used in clinical assessment of posture: normal posture, function-

Table 3. Posture terminology

	Possible synonyms	Synonyms to be avoided in scientific texts
1. Normal Posture	Normal posture Suitable posture Sound posture Regular posture	Good posture Beautiful posture Correct posture
2. Functional postural abnormality	Defective posture Unsuitable posture False posture Postural defects Functional postural disorders Functional postural damage (reversible postural damage)	Poor posture Unaesthetic posture
3. Structural postural abnormality	Morbid, pathologic posture Fixed postural deformities Structural postural abnormalities (irreversible postural damage)	Bad posture

Table 4. Postural performance

1. Full (normal) postural performance	Efficient, sound posture; normal, efficient, functional postural pattern
2. Postural weaknesses (postural insufficiency)	Weak, unstable posture; defective, incompetent, unsuitable, functional postural pattern
3. Postural degeneration (severe postural insufficiency)	Inefficient posture; pathologic, inefficient, postural pattern

Table 5. Normal posture

Structural characteristics	Physiologic, harmonious S-curves of the vertebral column (physiologic normal lordosis of the cervical and lumbar sections of the spine, and kyphosis of the thoracic section of the spine). Normal structural arrangement and position of the head, pectoral girdle, thorax, pelvis, extremities. Optimal line of gravity in normal, standing posture.
Functional characteristics	Normal harmonious postural pattern, retention of appropriate stable balance with minimal expenditure of energy, without compensatory postural effort by muscles and ligaments or correction of abnormal joint position.
Clinical importance	Sound posture Complete load-bearing and performance capabilities.

al postural abnormalities, and structural postural abnormalities. In functional assessment the terms full postural performance, postural insufficiency (postural weakness), and postural degeneration are used (Tables 3–4).

There is a continual transition from normal posture to functionally defective posture to real pathological postural disorders. Classification, particularly in office practice, is not always easy since it depends primarily on clinical experience, which is very subjective. Our remarks are primarily concerned with normal posture (habitual posture). The problematic change from a relaxed posture to a posture "at attention" will not be discussed. Normal posture is extremely difficult to define. However, it is certainly characterized structurally by appropriately developed physiological curves of the vertebral column. The normal form of kyphosis and lordosis is *functionally* supported in an upright position with a minimum of postural effort and without additional compensatory work by the muscles and ligaments of the back, trunk, pelvis, or lower limbs (Table 5). The person in question is said to have a "structurally and functionally efficient posture" (Matthiass 1966). Normal posture therefore requires not only a physiologic S-shaped vertebral column, but also normal arrangement of the remaining postural structures (thorax, pelvis, extremities, etc.). To be able to work efficiently, the same holds true for the functional dynamic postural elements. In normal standing posture the body is a perpendicular structure (Fig. 1). In the frontal plane, the optimal line of gravity falls from the head along the line of the spinous processes to the rima ani and between both feet to the ground. In the sagittal plane, the optimal line of gravity falls from the tip of the mastoid process, somewhat behind or along the cervical vertebrae, from approximately T-1 to T-2, in front of the thoracic spine, from L-1 behind the lumbar spine and then through the base of the sacrum at the level of the promontorium. It meets the hip joint either exactly at the axis of rotation or slightly behind it between the femoral head and the sacrum. It subsequently falls slightly in front of the knee joint and markedly in front of the pivot of the ankle joint. The pelvis is horizontal and its anterior angle of inclination is on the average 12° (Taillard 1964). Since so many varied forms may fall within the scope of normal posture, one must always remember that the form must be basically sound. It should require only a small amount of energy expenditure to maintain stable balance.

Functional postural abnormalities represent intermediary stages between normal posture and structural pathologic abnormalities. They are characterized by marked, permanent deviations from the normal postural form. However, they are not yet fixed structurally, but are functionally adjustable and can be actively corrected (Table 6). Functional postural abnormalities are primarily an indication of physiologic disorders, particularly functional deviations from the normal form. They must never be defined as pathologic, but may be *potentially pathologic.* They always require greater demands on postural performance since the curves of the vertebral column are no longer of correct size. However, increased postural performance is usually impossible, since functional postural abnormalities practically always involve postural insufficiency, and in fact they are usually even caused by this inadequacy. If functional postural abnormalities are not treated, i.e., functionally corrected, or if muscular compensation and postural performance are insufficient, it is impossible to prevent a transition to pathologic, permanently fixed, structural postural abnormalities. *Round-back, hollow-back, functional flat-back,* and *scoliotic posture without torsion* are included in functional abnormalities of posture.

Table 6. Functional postural abnormalities

Structural characteristics	Marked, permanent, purely functional deviations from the physiological S-shape of the vertebral column which are adjustable and correctible. Forms: Round-back (hyperkyphosis). Hollow-back (hyperkyphosis and hyperlordosis). Functional flat-back (lordosis of the thoracic spine and kyphosis of the cervical and lumbar spine). Scoliotic posture (without torsion). Often combined with additional deviations of other elements of the postural system (mainly the pectoral girdle, shape of the thorax, and position of the pelvis). Abnormal line of gravity in a normal standing posture.
Functional characteristics	Defective, incorrect, postural pattern. Usually combined with, or caused by, postural insufficiency. Abnormalities require increased compensatory postural effort, which is often not achieved.
Clinical importance	Conditionally pathologic, functional variations of posture. Strong tendencies to develop into pathologic abnormalities. Decreased load-bearing capacity and performance. Can be well treated functionally and therapeutically and is quite correctible ("preparation of normal postural pattern").

Table 7. Structural postural abnormalities

Structural characteristics	Pathologic deviations from the normal S-shape of the vertebral column. These deviations are pronounced, permanently fixed, and caused by structural abnormalities. Forms: kyphosis, lordosis, pathologic fixed flat-back (pathologic stretched straight posture), structural torsion, scoliosis, gibbus. Usually combined with additional functional and structural deviations in the rest of the postural system. Abnormal line of gravity in normal standing posture.
Functional characteristics	Pathologic, incorrect postural pattern. May be, but is not necessarily, combined with postural insufficiency. Necessary compensatory postural activity causes a permanent increase in expenditure of energy.
Clinical importance	Pathologic propensity for painful, functional degeneration, unsatisfactory postural performance leading to secondary degenerative changes. Load-bearing capacity and postural performance depend on the possibilities for functional compensatory support. The abnormalities are little, if at all, correctible from a functional therapeutic point of view, but postural performance and functional postural pattern may be improved.

In contrast to functional abnormalities, deviant curves of the vertebral column found in structural abnormalities of posture are fixed and are no longer correctible by functional means (Table 7). They are in fact actual pathologic postural abnormalities. A clinical distinction is made between the following structural abnormalities of the vertebral column: pathologic kyphosis and lordosis, pathologically fixed spinal extension, true structural scoliosis with torsion, and also gibbus. Structural postural abnormalities do not necessarily result in functional failure of posture. In fact, the better the functional efficiency, the greater is the adaptability and compensatory effect in these pathologic structural abnormalities. One can therefore fully understand why, for example, the thoracic kyphosis of Scheuermann disease does not cause the slightest trouble for an athlete with strong muscles. Conversely, all structural abnormalities of the vertebral column are empirically predisposing factors to premature secondary degenerative changes in the region of the vertebral column.

Tables 5 to 7 illustrate the varied, clinical distinctions between functional and structural abnormalities of posture. Functional postural abnormalities and pathologic structural abnormalities are always unsuitable. They undoubtedly lead to an incorrect postural pattern and require increased postural performance. Every functional and structural abnormality of the vertebral column is accompanied by disorders in other areas of body posture. Postural abnormalities may even be caused by these disorders which considerably broadens the need for therapy.

Posture as a Terminological Problem

In reviewing the literature, one is struck by the many different terms and definitions used in describing posture. Consequently there is a pressing need for a uniform terminology which is not open to misinterpretation. This should not be considered paltry word-quibbling. In our opinion, it is particularly important to make a clear distinction between functional postural abnormalities and pathologic, fixed, structural abnormalities of posture. This is particularly important for therapeutic reasons, since considerably different methods of treatment are required for these two groups of postural disorders, particularly if physiotherapy is used. The physiotherapist aims at producing an efficient postural pattern in patients with functional postural abnormalities. When irreversible structural changes are present, i.e., real fixed abnormalities, one must concentrate on increasing *postural performance*. Tables 3 and 5–7 summarize postural nomenclature used in our clinic, where mainly functional treatment is provided for postural disorders (Wagenhäuser 1968, 1977). Our nomenclature also corresponds with that used by many other authors. Synonyms, which are better avoided in scientific texts, are also cited.

In our opinion, the terms "kyphotic tendency" and "lordotic tendency" should be used to describe the physiologic curves of the vertebral column. The terms "kyphosis" and "lordosis" should define only fixed, permanent, pathologic formal anomalies of the vertebral column. Güntz (1957) and Hauberg (1958) define kyphosis as a permanent, abnormal increase in the curvature of the vertebral column or a specific section of the vertebral column, with dorsal convexity. They define lordosis as a permanent, pathologic curvature of the vertebral column with abnormally increased ventral convexity. Hauberg states that these terms should emphasize the irreversible, pathologic process, and that it therefore would be meaningful to talk of normal posture as "physiologic thoracic kyphosis, cervical or lumbar lordosis" respectively. In our opinion, the terms "lordotic tendency" and "kyphotic tendency" emphasize the functional meaning. It should be made clear that the term *scoliosis* should only be used for true, structural, torsional scoliosis (Lindemann 1958; Scheier 1967). The expression "(functional) scoliotic (inclination)" is used for purely functional deviations in the frontal plane, e.g., in cases of frontal pelvic inclination or nucleus pulposus hernias. In our opinion, there is an essential distinction between the terms kyphosis and round-back. In order to distinguish it strictly from fixed pathologic kyphosis, the term "round-back" should be used exclusively to mean a functional postural abnormality (functional, thoracic hyperkyphotic tendency). Again, such terminological differentiation is important both to determine the kind of therapy needed and in particular to evaluate and compare clinical statistics and epidemiologic studies (Wagenhäuser 1969, 1977)

Unfortunately, the term "good posture" has been used more and more instead of the term "normal posture". Similarly, functional and structural abnormalities of posture are often summarized indiscriminately as "bad posture". In our opinion, the expressions "bad" or "good" posture should be avoided in scientific texts as they are not used in other medical fields. They are also too easily associated with purely psychological or even moral values. No internist would refer to a "normal" cardiopulmonary condition as a "good heart" or "good lungs". The terms "good joint" or "good joint condition" are used just as infrequently in orthopaedics and rheumatology. The expressions "beautiful" and "correct" posture are similarly more suitable for literary usage. There is no doubt that normal posture is aesthetically beautiful. However, it is even more difficult to establish norms for aesthetically beautiful posture than for physically normal posture, as it is well-known that ideals of beauty change practically with every generation. Unlike the term "suitable posture", the expression "correct posture" is too closely connected with etiquette and customs of social behavior to be of scientific use. Considering all difficulties in defining the exact parameters of normal posture, we consider the term "suitable posture" despite, or even because of its somewhat indefinite scope, to be totally apt for practical and theoretical scientific usage.

Posture as a Psychological Problem

A summary of the controversial aspects of posture would be incomplete without a few brief sentences on its problematic psychological aspects. We have already pointed out that man's total psychological attitude is an essential element of total human posture. We agree with Schede that posture is an expression of the total psychosomatic aspects of a person and a measure of his strength. Routine daily clinical experience has shown that physical posture and mental attitude are closely connected. They have a reciprocal effect on each other. Unfortunately, compared with physical orthotherapy, the psychological aspects of orthotherapy are all too frequently completely neglected. Habitual psychological attitude can often be directly diagnosed from habitual physical posture. A frame of mind characterized by joy, happiness, success, self-reliance, trust, and confidence produces upright posture with its corresponding postural pattern. Conversely, grief, conflict, depression, failure and inferiority complexes have exactly the opposite effect and produce habitually defective postural patterns, of which stooping and a bowed-down stance are the most evident. A confident psychological background provides a good basis for sound postural performance. Insecurity favors the development of an uncertain, weak physical posture. Any layman can distinguish between the posture of an apathetic invalid and that of a graceful ballet dancer. This only touches the surface of the problem.

In clinical practice the relations between psychological phenomena and physical posture are not always so obvious, opening a wide field of study for modern psychosomatic medicine. It is of particular value for postural disorders in young people. There is no doubt that numerous known factors of modern civilization (mainly poor sitting habits and lack of physical exercise) work against the desired development of normal posture. However, Weintraub (1972) points out that psychosomatic damage to posture is indeed more frequent than is generally assumed, particularly among young people who experience marked growth acceleration and concomitant early onset of puberty. Stress caused by the incongruity of extrinsic physical appearance and intrinsic intellectual maturity manifests itself in specific postural disorders. Weintraub adroitly states: "These young people cannot keep up with their growth. They are bowed down by internal and external demands of premature bodily development." Postural degeneration of many adults harmed by the effects of civilization, demonstrates their inability to cope with their own personal fate and represents the intrinsic and extrinsic breakdown of posture under the weight of mental and physical burdens. Long ago, *Homo technicus* lost natural man's graceful, flexible, resistant, and supple posture, perfect in motion or at rest (Fig. 3a). However, not only factors of technical civilization have partly produced and partly threatened man's laborious acquisition of erect posture. Cultural development and related social etiquette and conduct throughout different historical epochs have without doubt created quite varied ideals of posture. We read Schede's inspired descriptions of classical sculptures as paragons of human posture with rather melancholic approval. Idols of postural perfection have changed with the passing of time. Velasquez depicted the small infanta Margarita in a splendid, yet severe, stiff posture "harness" composed of precious silk and soft fur. He aptly expressed the harsh postural Spanish court etiquette of the seventeenth century (Fig. 3b). Hardly any room is left for genuine, natural, human posture. We begin to feel compassion for the lovely, soft-faced child with her timid rather than regal eyes and the barely controlled lips which would rather smile.

Today's youth cannot complain of being forced into unnaturally rigid posture (Fig. 3c). The days of "Frederick, stand up straight, or you won't get into the army" are long gone. Frederick would rather accentuate his sloppy posture to escape from the physical and psychological demands of military service. Contemporary youths attribute their behavior and posture to "being cool", a typical modern adjective. Is this a change or a breakdown in postural form? Medicine will have to explore the physical and psychological aspects of this new crisis in human evolution.

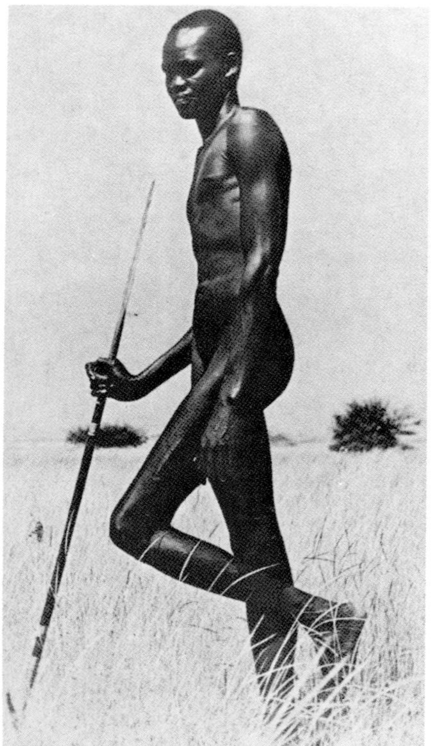

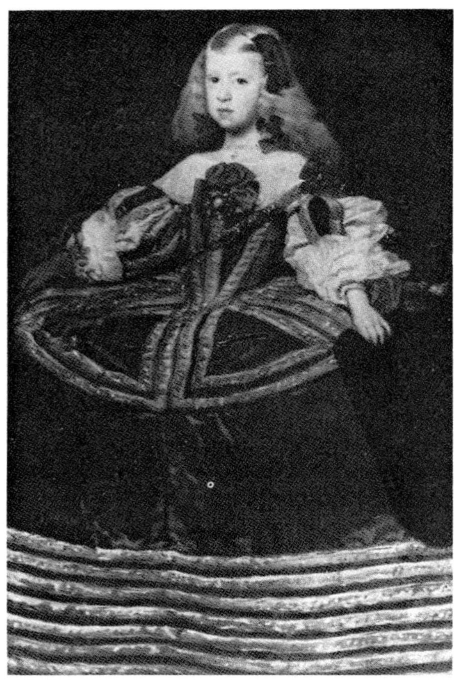

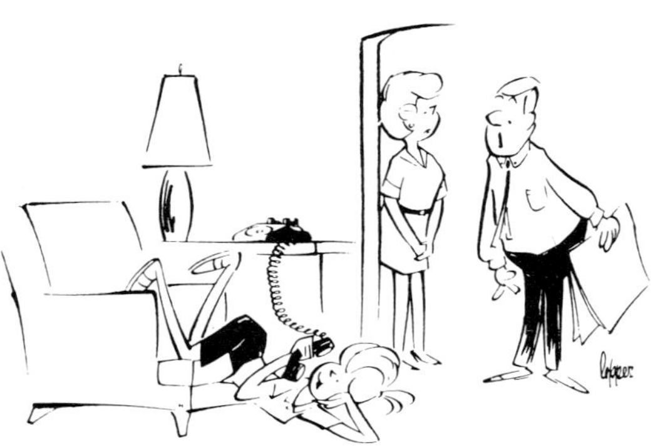

Fig. 3a–c. Markedly different ideals of "perfect" posture were created throughout history by cultural development and social rules and conduct related to it. **b** The rigid posture of the infanta Margarita. **c** "How tall is she now? I've not seen her standing upstraight for two years"

References

Benninghoff A, Goerttler K (1968) Lehrbuch der Anatomie des Menschen, Bd I. Urban & Schwarzenberg, Munich

Güntz F (1957) Die Kyphose im Jugendalter. Hippokrates, Stuttgart

Hauberg G (1958) Kyphosen und Lordosen. In: Handbuch der Orthopädie, Bd II. Thieme, Stuttgart, p 108

Leger W (1959) Die Form der Wirbelsäule. Enke, Stuttgart

Lindemann K (1958) Skoliosen. In: Hohmann G, Hackenbroch M, Lindemann K (eds) Handbuch der Orthopädie, Bd II. Thieme, Stuttgart, p 160

Lippert H (1970) Probleme der Statik und Dynamik von Wirbelsäule und Rückenmark. In: Trostdorf E, Stender HS (eds) Wirbelsäule und Nervensystem. Thieme, Stuttgart

Matthiass HH (1966) Reifung, Wachstum und Wachstumsstörungen des Haltungs- und Bewegungsapparates im Jugendalter. Karger, Basel Freiburg New York

Portmann A (1969) Biologische Fragmente zu einer Lehre vom Menschen, 3rd edn. Schwabe, Basel

Schede F (1969) Grundlagen der körperlichen Erziehung. Enke, Stuttgart

Scheier H (1967) Prognose und Behandlung der Skoliose. Thieme, Stuttgart

Steindler A (1955) Kinesiology. Thomas, Springfield

Taillard W (1964) Die Klinik der Haltungsanomalien. In: Belart W (ed) Die Funktionsstörungen der Wirbelsäule. Huber, Bern Stuttgart

Wagenhäuser FJ (1968) Bewegungsdiagnostik der Wirbelsäule in ihrer Gesamtheit und in ihren Regionen. In: Junghans H (ed) Die Wirbelsäule in Forschung und Praxis, Bd XI. Hippokrates Stuttgart

Wagenhäuser FJ (1969a) Z Praev Med 14:157

Wagenhäuser FJ (1969b) Die Rheumamorbidität. Eine klinisch-epidemiologische Untersuchung. Huber, Bern Stuttgart Vienna

Wagenhäuser FJ (1973) Die Haltungsstörungen der Wirbelsäule. In: Kaganas G, Müller W, Wagenhäuser FJ (eds) Vertebragene Syndrome. Karger, Basel. Fortbildk Rheumat, vol 2, pp 37–57

Wagenhäuser FJ (1977) Epidemiology of postural disorders in young people. In: Wagenhäuser FJ, Fehr K, Huskisson EC, Wilhelmi E (eds) Rheumatological research and the fight against rheumatic diseases in Switzerland. Monograph 1 Eular bulletin

Weintraub A (1972) Psychosomatik des Weichteilrheumatismus – therapeutische Konsequenzen in Kur und Praxis. Z Rheumaforsch 31:273

Translation from the German: Wagenhäuser FJ (1973) Das Problem der Haltung. Orthopäde 2: 128–139 © Springer Verlag 1973

Early Diagnosis of Osteonecrosis by Functional Bone Investigation

P. Ficat

Osteonecrosis is essentially a vascular disease. Death of bone tissue is nearly always the result of decreased blood supply or of insufficient circulation. Therefore, investigation of these two factors is a fundamental element in studying its pathology.

Classification of Osteonecrosis

In cooperation with Arlet (Ficat and Arlet 1977), we have proposed a four-stage classification with increased severity based on radiologic aspects:

Stage I (preradiologic stage)

The radiograph is normal or shows only slight osteoporosis. Clinically the hip may be asymptomatic, or it can be painful and its mobility slightly restricted. This stage may last for several months. Therefore hip pain with limitation of motion and without radiologic findings could be the first sign of osteonecrosis, and one should consider functional investigation of the bone to establish its presence.

Stage II

Joint line and femoral head contour are still normal, but cancellous bone changes are present. They may appear as: diffuse or partially spotty osteoporosis; sclerosis; mixed with spotty sclerosis.

Stage III

The joint line remains normal, but the contour of the head is interrupted. Further collapse results in sequestration.

Stage IV

The width of the joint line is decreased, and it begins to flatten. Extensive joint destruction is present, caused by osteonecrosis and by subsequent arthrosis.

Detection of the disease during its early stages (I, II) in order to prevent the irreversible lesions of later stages (III, IV) remains a problem. Radiographs of stages I and II are of no help in making a diagnosis. For this reason, we have developed a new diagnostic method that we call functional bone investigation. It makes the study of intraosseous circulation and several other parameters of bone metabolism possible.

Materials and Methods

Functional Bone Investigation

For investigative purposes a trochar of 3 mm diameter is driven into the trochanteric area of the femur with a mallet to insure a watertight seal at the lateral cortex. The trochar is connected with a tube to a pressure transducer coupled to a recording device. The tube is filled with heparinized normal saline solution (Fig. 1). The first step of the investigation is the recording of intraosseous pressure 5 min after trochar insertion. Usually, this basic pressure is below 30 mm Hg. Mean values of 42.3 ± 6.8 ($p \leq 0.01$) are found in osteonecrosis (Figs. 2, 3). Intraosseous injection of 5 ml normal saline solution does not produce pain. Intraosseous pressure increase is transient or nonexistent. This stress test is positive if pressure rises more than 10 mm Hg or if elevated values persist for more than 5 min.

The second step of the investigation consists of a transosseous venogram with 10 ml of a contrast medium injected through the trochar. Normally, rapid filling of the four ex-

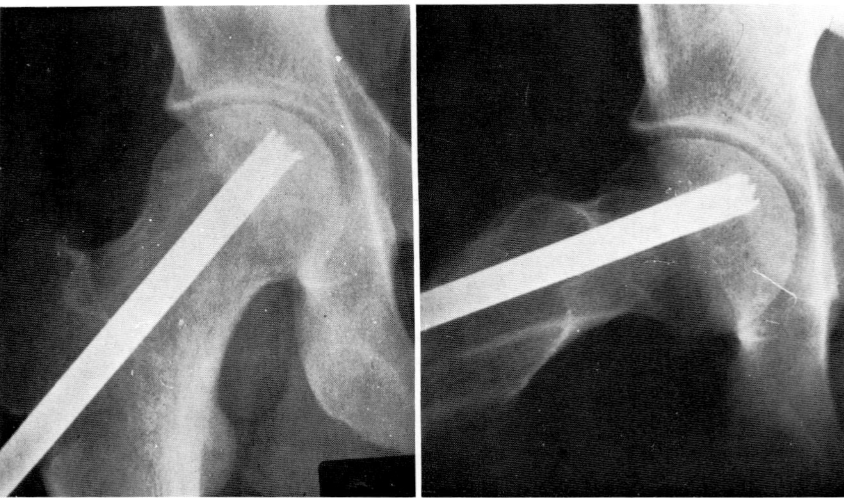

Fig. 1. Correct trochar position in the A.P. and lateral view

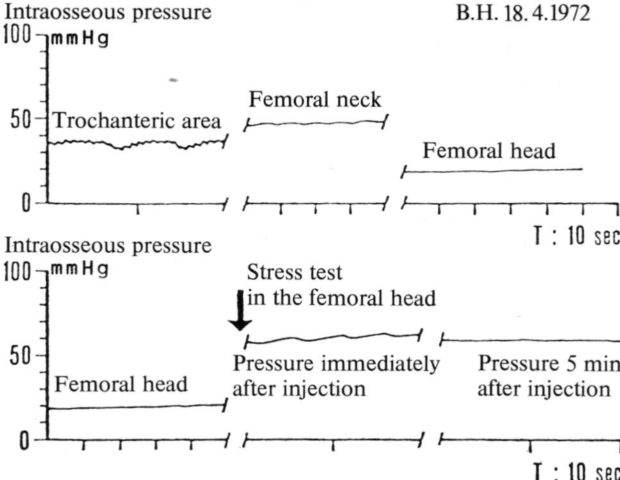

Fig. 2. Intraosseous pressure: Trochanteric area 35 mm Hg, femoral neck 45 mm Hg, femoral head 19 mm Hg. Positive stress test in the femoral head: 75 mm Hg, 5 min after trochar insertion

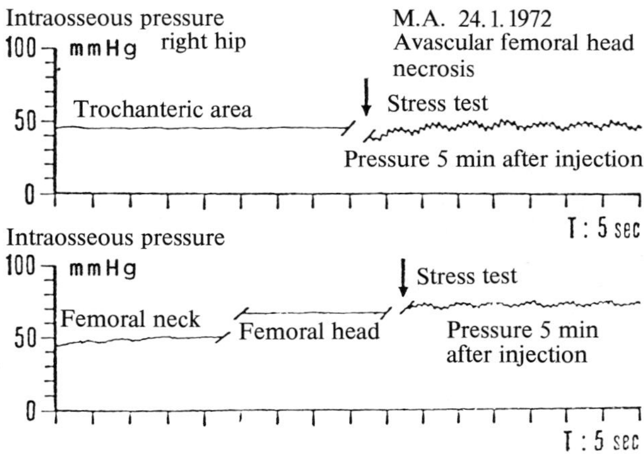

Fig. 3. Intraosseous pressure: Trochanteric area 45 mm Hg, femoral neck 45 mm Hg, femoral head 55 mm Hg. Stress test negative in trochanteric area, slightly positive in the femoral head (posttraumatic osteonecrosis)

traosseous main veins that drain the femoral region is noted. Radiographs are obtained immediately after injection and 5 and 10 min later. The entire intraosseous contrast material should be cleared after 5 min. Pathologic venograms show no or minimal filling of the extraosseous veins, mainly of v. circumflexa and v. ischiatica, and diaphyseal reflux of the contrast medium to a level below the lesser trochanter. Contrast medium stasis can be observed on the 5 min postinjection film (Figs. 4, 5, 6).

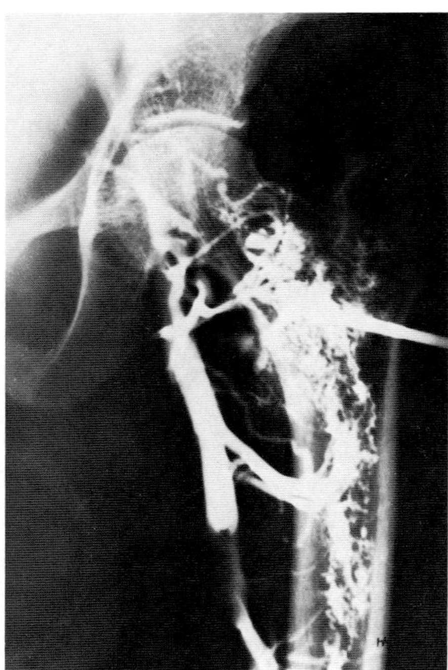

Fig. 4. Obvious reflux into the diaphysis in osteonecrosis of stage I

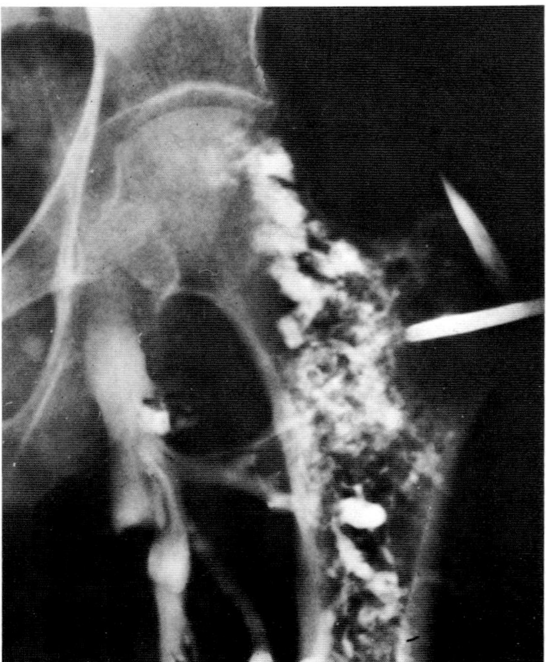

Fig. 5. Stage I osteonecrosis. Venous drainage of the hip is absent. Reflux into diaphysis and even into femoral neck and head. Marked difference as compared to the appearance of a normal hip on standard radiographs

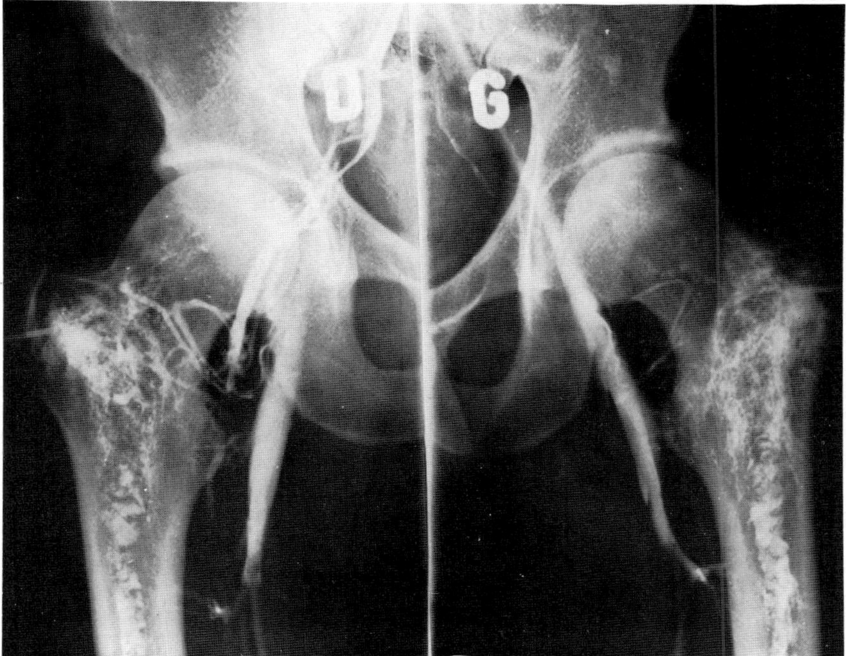

Fig. 6. Stage II osteonecrosis, bilateral venogram. Filling defect of the venae ischiaticae and reflux into the diaphysis

These two steps cover the hemodynamic phase of the investigation. It can be performed either in the trochanteric area or, if it should be negative there, in the area of the femoral head. We known from experience that we can speak of a syndrome of stasis and ischemia when the following are found:

Basic intraosseous pressure >30 mm Hg
Stress test >10 mm Hg
Filling defects in one or more efferent vessels
Diaphyseal reflux
Metaphyseal stasis

Scintigraphy

Increased uptake will usually be seen in the scintigram. This only means that the head of the femur is pathologically involved, but it is not pathognomonic for osteonecrosis. Scintigraphy can be negative in the presence of a positive functional bone investigation.

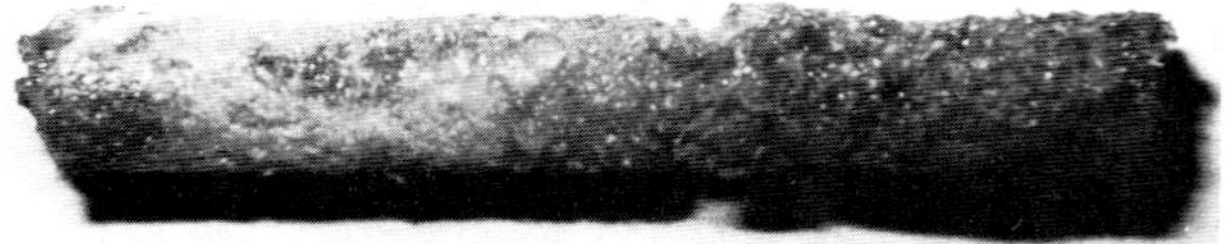

Fig. 7. Gross specimen of a cylindrical core biopsy. The head portion is on the left side of the picture (same patient is in Fig. 4)

Oxygen Saturation

Measuring oxygen saturation is of greater importance as it indisputably correlates with the intramedullary pressure of the trochanteric area. Average oxygen saturation values are $88.32 \pm 1.5\%$ ($p \leq 0.001$) in the presence of osteonecrosis of the femoral head. It is probably caused by lack of oxygen utilization. It has to be mentioned that we were unable to measure oxygen saturation in the femoral head or its sequestrated portion.

Temperature

Temperature measurements in cases of osteonecrosis revealed values below 36 °C. They are lower in the femoral head than in the trochanteric area. The lowest values were found in the sequestrum.

All these parameters enable us to explore a wide field of intraosseous circulation disturbances and their mutual metabolic relation. But it is also necessary to investigate their effects on bone marrow and on the trabecular system. Only this knowledge will confirm the diagnosis with certitude.

The last step of investigation is to obtain a core biopsy from the femoral head and neck. A special tool permits removal of a bone cylinder that suffices for histologic examination (Fig. 7). Under normal circumstances, spongy bone is a mixture of hematopoietic and fatty bone marrow situated between trabeculae which contain live osteocytes. In cases of osteonecrosis, several types of alterations will be observed.

Type I. Disappearance of the hematopoietic elements from bone marrow, dissociation of fat cells by stasis and edema, hemorrhage, xanthomatosis.

Type II. Fat cell necrosis and complete disorganization of fatty marrow, which appears to be fragmented into a new fine-meshed network. This is called reticular eosinophilic necrosis (Arlet). Occasionally one finds complete homogenization of the bone marrow (Fig. 8).

Type III. Total necrosis of bone marrow and trabecular system. Osteocytes have disappeared, the lacunae are empty and frequently enlarged. Trabeculae appear to be abnormal and are of pale color. Microfractures, washed-out margins, and fissures at the cement lines are present (Fig. 9).

Type IV. Total necrosis combined with fibrosis of the intramedullary canal and new bone apposition on necrotic trabeculae, representing an attempt to regenerate.

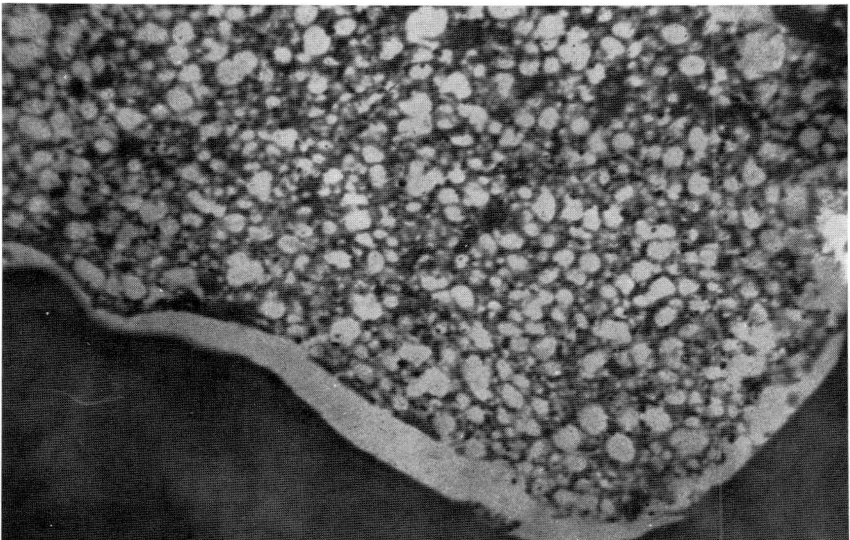

Fig. 8. Reticular eosinophilic necrosis of the bone marrow with fragmentation of the fat cells (type II)

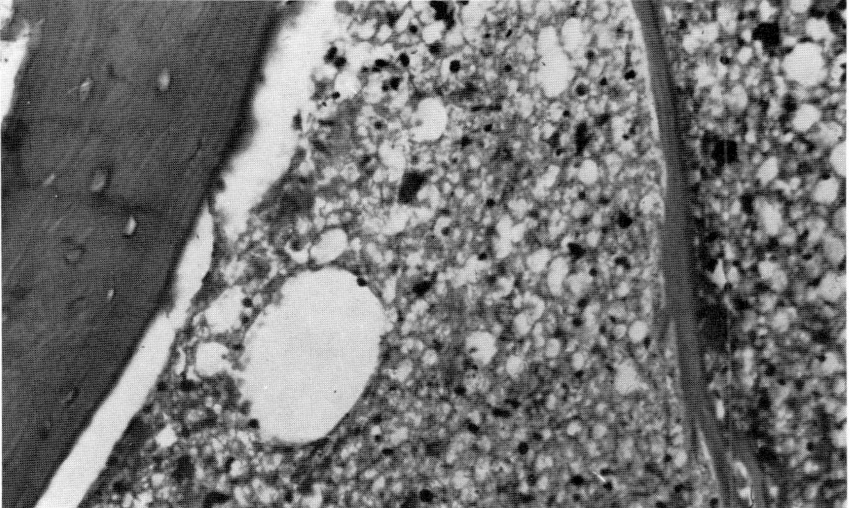

Fig. 9. Osteonecrosis type III. Total necrosis of fatty marrow and trabeculae

Discussion

Our method of hemodynamic bone investigation is very exact. In 99% of cases it permits diagnosis of stages I and II of hips suspected of being affected by osteonecrosis. It presupposes the systematic performance of every step of functional bone investigation. *Best* results are obtained during the early stages of disease. Normal or lower than normal intraosseous pressure may be found in stage III. This is probably caused by communications

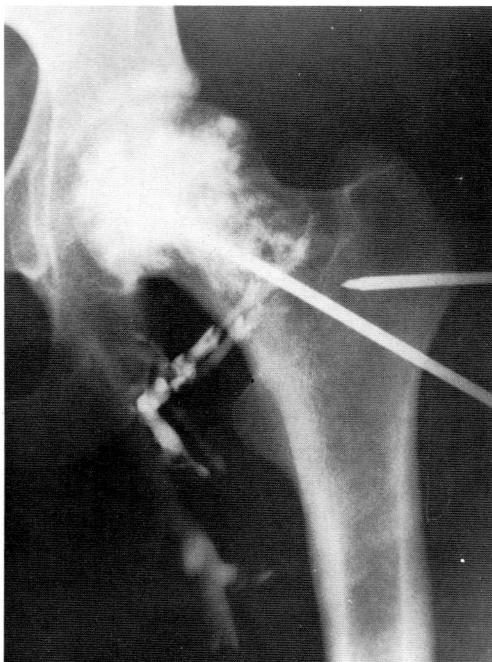

Fig. 10. Femoral head venogram in a case of ischemic coxopathy. Obvious stasis 15 min after injection

between bone and the joint space, whose pressure is always below normal or even negative. For the same reason, a venogram can turn into an arthrogram.

Data obtained from functional bone investigation allow differentiation between osteonecrosis and arthrosis. In arthrosis intramedullary pressure is less elevated than in osteonecrosis. In arthrosis mean values of 28.8% ± 4 (p ≦ 0.01) were found. The stress test is positive in 47%, compared with 77% in cases of osteonecrosis. The venogram is normal in coxarthrosis caused by hip dysplasia. In cases of primary osteoarthrosis, it is pathologic. In contrast to osteonecrosis, we found that hemodynamic disturbances corresponded to the amount of joint destruction. Scintigram uptake is less in arthrosis, as previously demonstrated by Crutchlow (1970) (hip) and Muheim and Bohne (1970) (knee). Mean oxygen saturation values of 79.5% ± 3.9 (p ≦ 0.001) are also diminished in cases of arthrosis, as compared to osteonecrosis.

Histologic examination of the bone core biopsy shows less extensive bone marrow necrosis in cases of arthrosis. These data enable us to identify a specific type of osteonecrosis, where collapse of the femoral head has not yet developed but, where in concordance with arthrosis, the joint space begins to diminish. The diagnosis of this type of osteonecrosis is impossible without functional bone investigation (Fig. 10).

There is no exact correlation between the histologic types and the radiologic stages. A radiologic stage I can show features of type III or IV. Similar differences were found when comparing intraosseous pressure and venogram, or clinical symptoms and radiograph.

The constant presence of circulatory disturbances during all stages of the disease and in particular during the early stages permit the description of an ischemic syndrome. It is the common denominator of all stages and of all etiologic forms. Its discovery in asymptomatic, radiologic normal hips that later develop clinical symptoms and histologic changes of ischemia implies that these abnormalities are important in the pathogenesis of osteonecrosis.

The remarkable uniformity of the disease in regard to symptoms, radiologic appearance, circulatory abnormalities, progression, anatomical location, and final outcome is in contrast to the multiplicity and variety of its presumed causes (trauma, steroid therapy, sickle cell anemia, Gaucher disease, caisson disease, arteritis, alcohol abuse, gout, hip dysplasia, thrombophlebitis, and lipoid metabolism disturbances). These facts imply the presence of a common pathogenic factor involving the intraosseous circulation.

The response of the bone marrow to ischemia is uniform, in spite of a great variety of noxious factors (mechanical interruption of circulation, either arterial or venous; arteriolar embolism; bone marrow proliferation; intramedullary fat hypertrophy; intravascular clotting from every cause). Stasis and edema increase intraosseous pressure and vascular resistance and decrease blood flow, causing a vicious circle. This process progresses slowly, finally resulting in necrosis and collapse of those bony portions that are most involved.

Each trabecular ring of cancellous bone acts as a channel for the proliferation of bone marrow and its vessels. Therefore osteonecrosis can be compared with other compartment syndromes.

This hypothesis is supported by the response to decompression as a result of the core biopsy. The biopsy is not only of histologic value. Its therapeutic effect can be observed by the rapid disappearance of pain and by the influence on the course of the disease and its final outcome. This has been proven by our statistical results.

Results

In a series of 131 cases, we can report long-term results (observation period of at least 5 years) in 108 cases of stages I and II. Of the remaining 23 cases without long-term observation, 5 died of nonrelated causes while the other 18 were followed for 1–3 years. A good result was found in 15 cases, a poor result in 3.

Ninety-nine patients (55 males, 44 females) had 108 observations of osteonecrosis. In 57 cases involvement of the right hip was noted, in 51 cases involvement of the left. Of the 27 patients with bilateral involvement, 9 were operated on both sides. Sixty-nine cases belonged to stage I, 39 to stage II. Nearly one-third of all cases were between ages 40 and 50. The time of follow-up was between 5 and 15 years (mean, 7.9 years).

Results were evaluated according to clinical criteria and the course of radiologic changes. Clinical results were good in 99 cases, but radiologic results were good in only 85 cases. In 23 (21.5%) cases, we observed radiologic deterioration; 9 (8.3%) were also clinical failures.

A second operation was performed in seven of the nine cases; four of them underwent a second core biopsy. In none of these patients was reappearance of osteonecrosis present. The reintervention was successful in two cases.

Radiologic deterioration can present as progressive narrowing of the joint space (17 cases). We call this condition ischemic coxopathy (seven cases of stage I, ten cases of stage II). It can also present as collapse of the femoral head (two cases of stage I, four cases of stage II).

Conclusions

Some authors reported the spontaneous development of stages I and II without confirmation by core biopsy. Marcus et al. (1973) observed hip osteonecrosis of stage II of our classification and called them silent hips. A collapse of the femoral head (stage III) occurred in two-thirds of their cases within 2 years. They operated on 11 hips, employing a technique similar to our own, and observed very good results in ten cases during reexaminations after 2–4 years.

Hungerford (1979) was able to follow 27 patients for more than a year. These patients had unilateral hip involvement; the other hip was radiologically normal and without clinical symptoms (stage 0). Ten of these patients had a normal functional bone investigation, 17 had either increased intraosseous pressure or a pathologic venogram, or both. Eleven of these 17 patients had a histologically proven osteonecrosis 10 days to 18 months later.

These reports corroborate our results. They show that the normal course of stages I and II of osteonecrosis leads to femoral head collapse in 66% of cases within the first 18 months.

In contrast, our 108 cases treated by cylinder bone core biopsy and followed for a mean period of 7.5 years developed collapse of the femoral head in only 5.5%. This difference is highly significant, and it proves the effectiveness of the core biopsy for the early stages of the disease. It is important to note that our series does not contain cases with kidney transplantations or dysbaric conditions.

In conclusion, we would like to state that early diagnosis, i.e., prior to the appearance of radiologic changes, is one of the most important advances in the treatment of osteonecrosis. Its diagnosis is based on functional bone investigation, as osteonecrosis is the response to vascular impairment of bone marrow circulation.

References

Crutchlow W (1970) Sr. 85 scintimetry of the hip in osteoarthritis and osteonecrosis. 109:803
Ficat P, Arlet J (1977) Ischémie et nécrose osseuses. Masson, Paris New York Barcelone Milan. English translation by Hungerford. Williams and Wilkins. Baltimore 1980. 1942.
Marcus ND, Eneking WF, Massam RA (1973) The silent hip in idiopathic aseptic necrosis. Treatment by bone grafting. J Bone Joint Surg [Am] 55:1351

Muheim G, Bohne WH (1970) Prognosis in spontaneous osteonecrosis of the knee. J Bone Joint Surg [Br] 52:605
Hungerford DS (1979) Bone marrow pressure, venography and core decompression in ischemic necrosis of the femoral head. Hip Society Meeting, Proceedings 1979, pp 218–237

Translation from the German: Ficat P (1980) Vasculäre Besonderheiten der Osteonekrose. Orthopäde 9:238–244 © Springer Verlag 1980

Early Diagnosis and Treatment of Ischemic Necrosis of the Femoral Head

D. S. Hungerford

A review of the literature would seem to indicate that ischemic necrosis of the femoral head (INFH) is growing in importance as a clinical entity. In 1962, Mankin and Brower found only 22 cases in the English literature, to which they added five of their own. Since then, series with more than 100 cases have been reported (Ficat et al. 1971; Merle d'Aubigné et al. 1965). In 1948, Chandler postulated that blockage of the posterolateral retinacular artery leads to infarction and eventual collapse of the anterolateral area of the femoral head. The typical X-ray picture supported that hypothesis in what appeared to be a wedge-shaped bone infarct (Fig. 1). This concept of "coronary disease of the hip" seemed almost self-evident and was widely accepted. Although this might be the case for post-traumatic INFH, a wide variety of other apparent etiologic associations, including

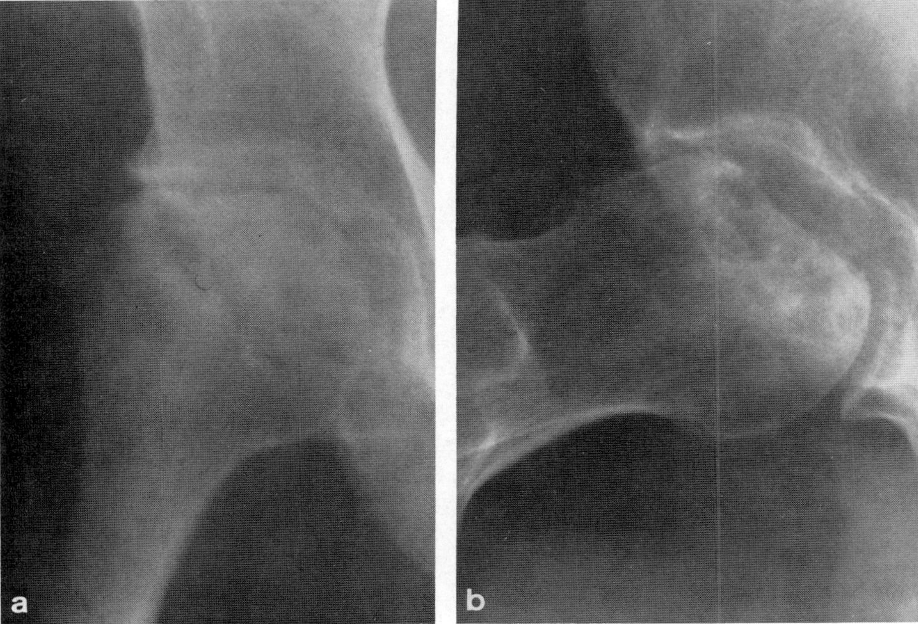

Fig. 1a, b. The typical anterolateral localization of the collapsing segment as seen on the **a** anteroposterior and **b** lateral X-ray of the hip certainly suggests an arterial wedge infarction

alcohol abuse (18), both endogenous and exogenous steroid excess (Cruess et al. 1968; Edstrom 1971; Harrington et al. 1971; Soloman 1973), connective tissues diseases, especially systemic lupus erythematosis (Dubois 1960; Zizic et al. 1980), gout, Gaucher's disease, and hemoglobinopathy (Dubois 1960), all have a similar morphological localization which would seem to transcend the simple mechanical involvement of a single artery. The mechanisms by which these diverse presumed etiologic associations produce such a similar clinical pattern have been the source of considerable controversy.

It is well known that the early phases of bone ischemia pass undetected by X-ray and may cause only minimal symptoms. The typical patient presents with a several week history of intermittent pain and a very short history of more severe pain, at which time the X-ray shows early evidence of collapse. Some patients, however, do have more severe symptoms in the preradiologic or early stage of the disease. Since most authors report a high incidence of eventual bilateral involvement, regardless of the suspected etiologic association with the exception of trauma, many patients presenting with a unilateral disease will develop signs and symptoms of involvement of the second side during the period of observation (Ficat et al. 1971; Hungerford and Zizic 1978; Merle d'Aubigne et al. 1968). This presents the treating physician with an opportunity to make the diagnosis on the second side prior to morphological failure of the femoral head.

Larsen (1938) appears to have been the first to have recognized an association between increasing bone marrow pressure (BMP) and bone necrosis, producing the latter experimentally. Serre and Simon (1961) were the first to apply intraosseous venography to the proximal femur in INFH and to discover an increase in BMP. Arlet and Ficat (1968) described increased BMP in 42 cases in the preradiologic stage of the disease. They correlated these discoveries with the histologic changes in the biopsy specimen. Since 1973 we have systematically been applying their techniques of BMP measurements, venography, and core decompression to the diagnosis and treatment of INFH (Hungerford 1975, 1979; Hungerford and Zizic 1978). The findings and results allow an insight into the pathogenesis of ischemia and necrosis of bone and also lay the foundation for an early detection and treatment system.

The Suspicious Hip

Each patient with the above-described possible etiologic associations and inexplicable hip pain or with definite INFH of the opposite hip should be regarded as a high-risk patient for developing bone necrosis. The clinical picture can be quite variable, with pain usually starting gradually and intermittently, but occasionally appearing with sudden onset. The symptoms are generally described as deep and throbbing in nature. Groin pain is the typical localization, but buttock, lateral hip, and midthigh pain are also compatible with the diagnosis. Clinical examination shows a painful limitation of movement, especially on forced internal rotation.

Unfortunately, we continue to see patients who had been assured they did not have INFH solely because the first X-ray was interpreted as negative. It must be understood that all cases of bone necrosis pass through a preradiologic stage, and that even the earliest radiologic changes indicate that the disease process has been in progress for some time. The fact that many patients have no symptoms or minimal symptoms during this preradiologic stage should not deter us from seeking to establish the diagnosis during this early phase of the disease when there is hope that its progression can be arrested or retarded.

Materials and Methods

The patients reported in this series were seen by the author at The Johns Hopkins Hospital, The Veterans Administration Hospital, and The Good Samaritan Hospital of Baltimore between January 1973 and June 1980. They had bone marrow pressure measurement and histologic confirmation of the disease. Most patients also had intramedullary venography. The presumed etiologic association for this series is shown in Table 1. The radiographic classification of INFH according to Arlet and Ficat has been found useful and relates specifically to both treatment category and prognosis (Table 2). The results of treatment are reported only for the precollapse stages of the disease.

Method of Study

Although it is possible to carry out BMP measurements under local anesthesia, most patients had the pressure measured at the time of a planned surgical intervention and under general or spinal anesthesia. Intramedullary venography is very painful, even in patients without INFH, and severely painful in patients with an already elevated BMP. Therefore, venography should never be carried out in the absence of either systemic analgesia and sedation or general anesthesia.

Measurement of BMP requires a watertight seal at the outer cortex and a closed system. It is not possible to measure BMP accurately with an open manometer system. A

Table 1. Clinical conditions associated with INFH

Clinical condition	Number of patients	Number of hips
Trauma	12	13
Steriod therapy (total)	63	104
Systemic lupus erythematosus	35	59
Rheumatoid arthritis	2	3
Renal transplant	10	15
Miscellaneous	16	27
Gaucher's disease	2	3
Alcohol abuse	39	62
Sickle cell disease	3	5
None (idiopathic)	9	12
Caisson's disease	2	4
Total	130	203

Table 2. Radiologic classification of ischemic necrosis of the femoral head (from Ficat and Arlet 1980)

	Stage	Joint-line	Femoral head contour	Trabeculae	Diagnosis by X-ray	Diagnosis by functional exploration of bone
Simple necrosis	I	N	N	N or very slight osteoporosis	Impossible	Hemodynamic-probable
	II	N	N	Osteoporosis mixed sclerosis/ porosis	Probable	Histo-pathological certain
Necrosis complicated by collapse	III	N	Flattened subchondral infraction, collapse	Sequestrum formation	Certain	Confirmation
	IV	Nar-rowed	Collapsed	Destruction of superior pole	Very difficult between arthrosis, flammatory arthritis, and necrosis	Heomdynamic insufficient combined biopsy necessary

N = Normal

2–3 mm trocar is inserted with a mallet through the softer lateral part of the greater trochanter into the intertrochanteric region at the base of the neck. The obturator of the trocar creates a small artifact within which the pressure is measured. The intraosseous trocar is filled retrograde with heparinized saline using a 8.9-cm spinal needle. The trocar is then connected to a pressure transducer by a semirigid polyethylene tubing such as is used in a cardiac catheterization laboratory. A three-way stopcock at the connecting point between the tubing and the trocar allows saline to be injected into the bone as a form of stress test while still maintaining a "closed" system. When the system is connected and the intraosseous artifact communicates with the pressure transducer, the recorded pressure rapidly rises to a plateau between 15 and 30 mm Hg (Fig. 2). The tracing reflects both arterial pulsations and undulation with respiration. If these are not seen, then the tip of the trocar either is not in bone or there is an obstruction somewhere in the system. Once the steady plateau has been reached, the BMP is remarkably stable over a long period of observation. It usually takes 2–3 min for this steady state to be achieved. This is referred to as the baseline pressure.

The injection of 5 ml isotonic saline intraosseously tests the capability of the vascular system within the bone to accept and discharge a fluid load. This is referred to as the "stress" test. Under normal circumstances bone is capable of handling this volume load without sustained elevation of BMP (Fig. 3). Any deviations from the resting pressure will normally return to the baseline within a few seconds. However, in the case of INFH a prolonged intraosseous hypertension is usually provoked. Our definition of abnormal

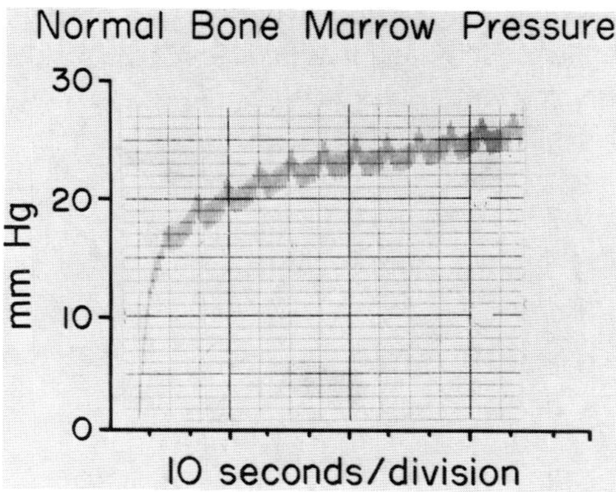

Fig. 2. The bone marrow pressure rapidly rises to a plateau between 20 mm Hg and 30 mm Hg. Pulse pressure and undulation with respiration are characteristic of the tracing (Hungerford 1979)

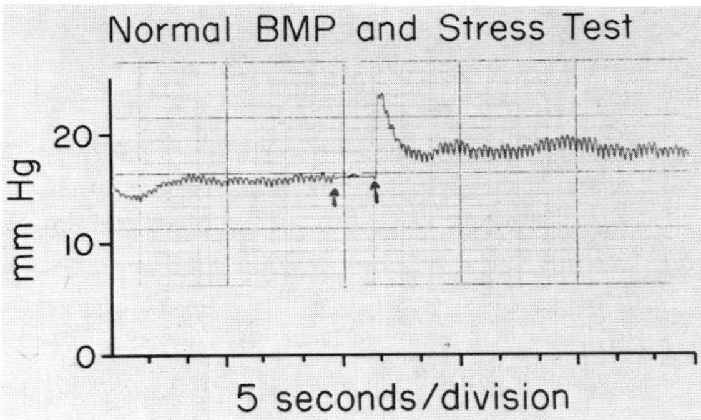

Fig. 3. After the tracing has stabilized, 5 ml isotonic saline are injected intraosseously (*arrows*). In normally vascularized bone, this stress test does not significantly elevate the marrow pressure

consists of a pressure rise of more than 10 mm Hg sustained for more than 5 min. The BMP after this 5-min period of observation is referred to as the stress test pressure. Finally, 8 ml renographin 60 is injected intraosseously. An AP radiograph is taken at the termination of injection and 5 minutes later.

Core Decompression

For those patients with symptoms or X-ray changes and in whom INFH is strongly suspected, a core biopsy is carried out. Through a short midlateral longitudinal incision centered over the proximal femoral metaphysis, the lateral metaphysis is exposed subperiosteally. Using a tapered reamer over a Steinmann pin, a 12–13 mm hole in the lateral cortex is created. Through this a hollow-core biopsy trocar is directed under biplane X-ray or image intensification control into the anterolateral segment of the femoral head. The specimen contains little artifact and is satisfactory for routine histology. The lateral gutter is drained, but not the core tract. Postoperatively, it is important to maintain the patient on protected weight-bearing with two crutches for 6 weeks to protect against fracture through the cortical window. It may be necessary to protect the patient for a much longer period to allow for stabilization of more advanced disease. Two patients with stage III disease who discarded their crutches prior to the 6 weeks sustained fractures through the cortical window. No patients sustained fractures after the 6 weeks.

Results

Bone marrow pressure measurements and intramedullary venograms were carried out with informed consent in patients having either surgical procedures not involving the hips or conditions not associated with INFH. The contralateral hip in patients with post-traumatic INFH were also considered as normal controls. All controls had normal physical examinations and negative radiographs of the hips and were asymptomatic referrable to the hip.

Normal BMP seldom rises above 30 mm Hg and never shows more than a 10 mm Hg increase in response to the stress test. Most controls showed a slight fall in BMP in response to the injection of saline intraosseously (see Fig. 3). The normal venogram demonstrates rapid filling of the extraosseous metaphyseal veins of the proximal femur with no evidence of diaphyseal reflux. Within 5 min most of the dye has been cleared from the bone (Fig. 4).

The BMP findings for patients with nontraumatic INFH in this series matched to the stage of the disease are reported in Table 3. It should be noted that the pressures are taken in the intertrochanteric region and not in the femoral head. This means that the BMP elevations are affecting more than that area to which radiographic changes are limited. Figure 5 gives an example of the BMP and stress test in a patient with the preradiologic stage of INFH (stage I). The intraosseous venogram in INFH shows poor filling of the main metaphyseal veins of the proximal femur and significant reflux. The 5-min film shows considerable intraosseous retention of the dye (Fig. 6).

The histologic findings in the later stages of INFH have been widely demonstrated and reveal extensive areas of necrosis and collapse involving primarily the anterolateral segment of the femoral head. However, the histologic changes in the early stages of bone necrosis have not been widely recognized. Subtle changes in bone marrow are the earliest histologic evidence of bone ischemia. The normal marrow contains relatively uniform-sized lipocytes with scattered foci of hematopoiesis (Fig. 7). In stage I INFH the marrow shows complete disappearance of hematopoiesis and a breakdown in the lipocyte pattern with fat-laden histiocytes (Fig. 8). Thickened trabeculae lined with osteoblasts may also be seen in stage I and early stage II (Fig. 9). In the later stages of the disease, the marrow changes have progressed to show extensive marrow fibrosis and trabecular hypertrophy with the center of the larger trabeculae devoid of osteocytes (Fig. 10).

We have always taken the opportunity to study the asymptomatic radiographically negative contralateral hip in patients presenting with unilateral INFH. Twenty-seven

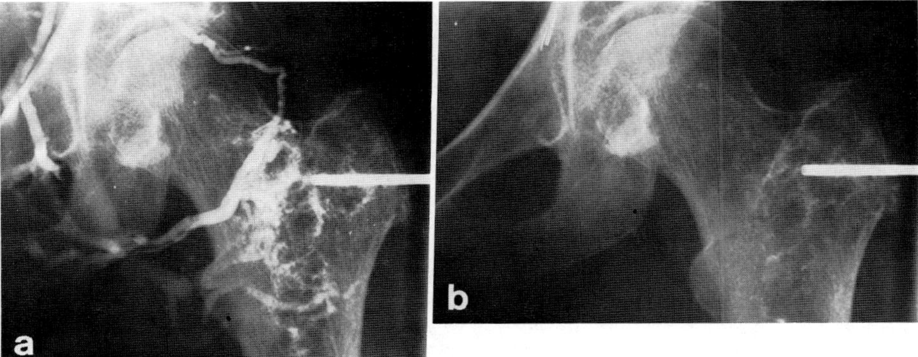

Fig. 4. a An injection of Renografin 60 intraosseously visualizes the proximal metaphyseal veins of the femur. **b** Five minutes after the injection, most of the dye has cleared the bone (Zizic et al. 1980)

Table 3. BMP findings in nontraumatic INFH

Stage	Number of hips	Baseline pressure[a]	Stress test[a]
I	22	34 (18–78)	62 (30–103)
II	26	54 (22–80)	68 (34–110)
III	142	48 (20–96)	59 (28–107)
Total	190	49 (18–98)	64 (28–110)
Controls	22	18 (3–38)[b]	18 (10– 28)

[a] Both baseline pressures and stress tests are significantly elevated compared to controls at P < 0.001, using one-way analysis of variance.

[b] Only one control had a baseline pressure greater than 30 mm Hg.

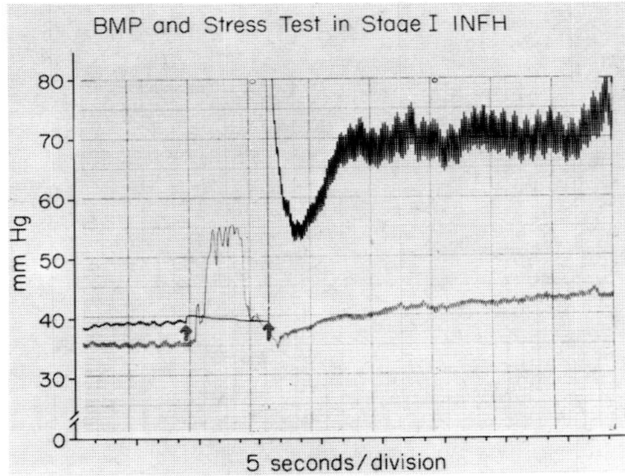

Fig. 5. Many patients with INFH will have an elevated baseline BMP (above 30 mm Hg). Most will have a dramatic increase of BMP with the stress test

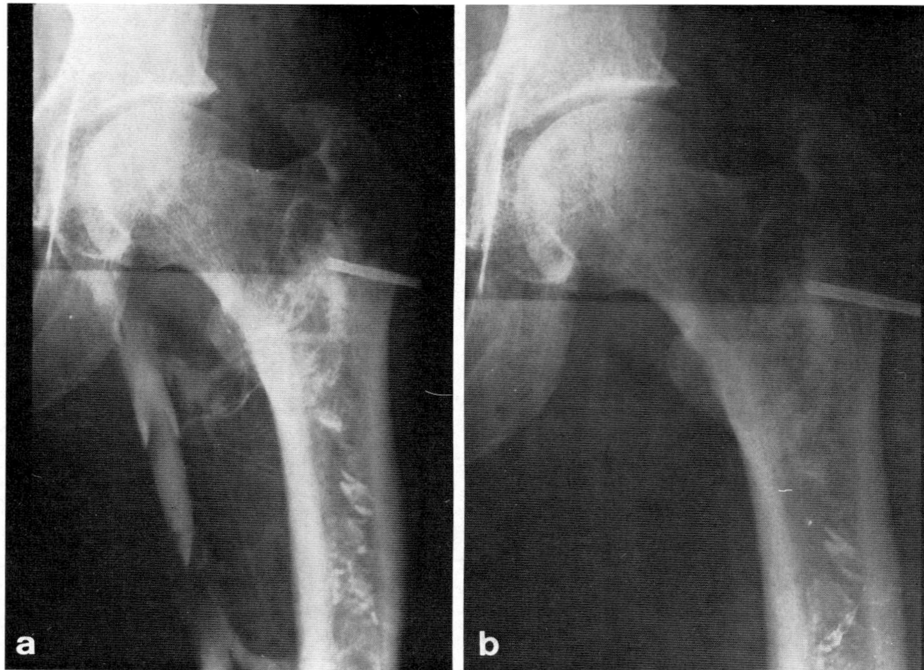

Fig. 6. The venogram in INFH shows **a** poor filling of diaphyseal veins and diaphyseal reflux and **b** considerable intraosseous retention of dye on the 5-min film (Hungerford 1979)

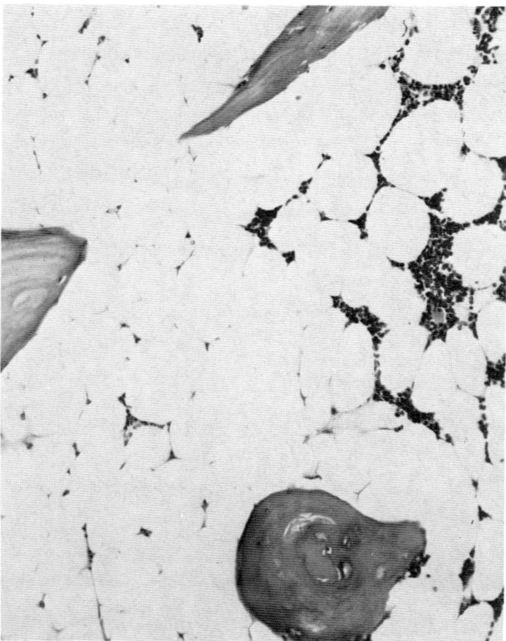

Fig. 7. Normal bone marrow from the proximal femur shows orderly, regular-sized lipocytes and a sprinkling of foci of hematopoiesis. ×175

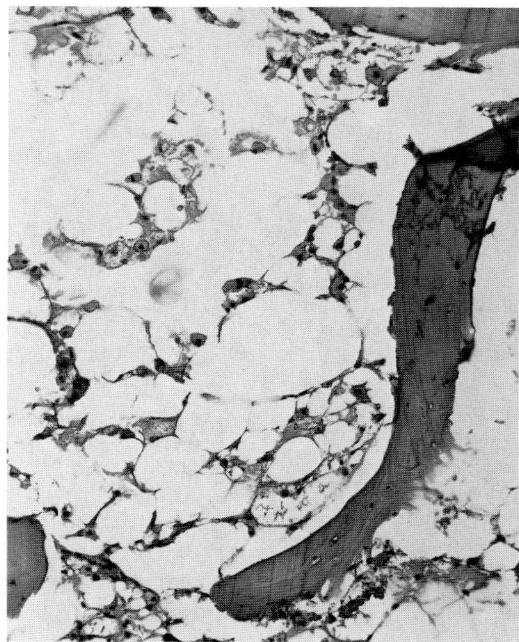

Fig. 8. Early marrow changes show a breakdown in the lipocytes with fat-laden histiocytes. ×175

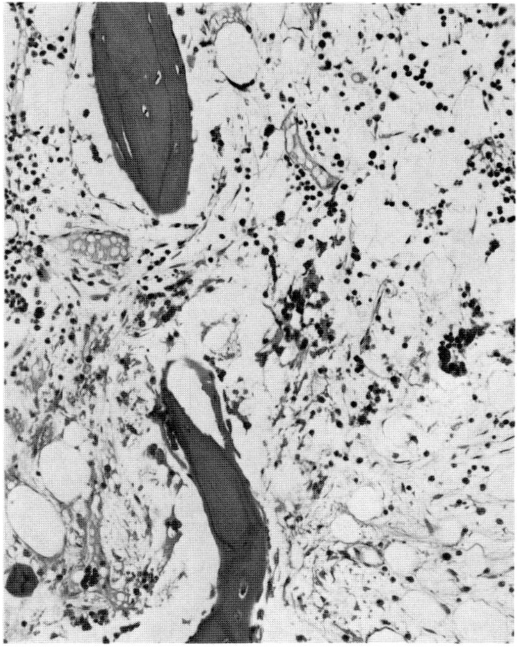

Fig. 9. Thickened, osteoblast-lined trabeculae, which still appear viable and are associated with marked marrow charges, may be evident even in stage I disease

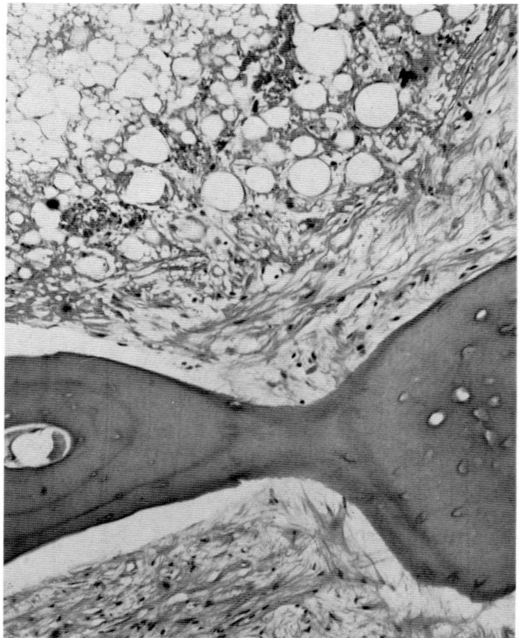

Fig. 10. Late disease with extensive marrow *and* trabecular changes

such patients have had BMP measurements, stress tests, and venograms carried out at the time of treatment of the symptomatic side. Bone marrow pressure and stress tests were normal in ten of these patients. With a minimum follow-up of 2 years, only one patient in this group has subsequently developed INFH. One year after her normal BMP study, this patient with systemic lupus erythematosus (SLE) had a flare-up of her disease, requiring additional high-dose steroid therapy. She developed symptomatic and radiologically evident INFH 6 months later, at which time the BMP findings were abnormal. Seventeen patients from this group had either elevated baseline pressures or abnormal stress tests at the time that they were studied. Thirteen have subsequently developed biopsy-proven INFH. Thus a preclinical group is identified in which elevated BMP heralds a high risk of developing symptomatic disease.

Creating a hole in the lateral femoral cortex in a patient with elevated BMP results in an immediate fall in intraosseous pressure. Patients with pain at rest report a decrease in symptoms in the immediate postoperative period, which is similar to that reported by patients with severe osteoarthrosis treated by medial displacement osteotomy. This diminution in symptoms appears to have lasting value only in the precollapse stage of INFH (stages I, II) (Ficat and Arlet 1968; Hungerford 1975; Hungerford and Zizic 1978). Although the results in stage II disease are not as predictable as in the precollapse stage, some patients may achieve prolonged palliation. Certainly core decompression for stage III disease cannot be enthusiastically recommended, but in certain patients who may be high risks for alternative measures of treatment, core decompression can offer palliation which, when coupled with some degree of protective weight-bearing, may offer symptomatic control for several years.

Table 4. Results of core decompression in INFH

Stage	Number of hips (patients)	No symptoms; no X-ray changes	X-ray progression	Further surgery	Follow-up in years (range)
I	18 (16)	16	2	1	5 (2.5–7.5)
II	23 (23)	16	7	4	4.2 (2.5–6.5)

Since core decompression appears to be most applicable for the early stages of disease, our results in stages I and II are reported here in some detail. Eighteen hips in 16 patients with stage I of INFH have been followed for $2^1/_2$–$7^1/_2$ years, with an average of 5 years (Table 4). Three patients were lost to follow-up after 3 years, but are included here according to their known status at last follow-up. Sixteen hips in 14 patients were asymptomatic and without X-ray evidence of progression. One patient required total hip replacement 14 months after core decompression because of progressive collapse of the femoral head. There were no operative or postoperative complications in this group. All patients were put on protective weight-bearing with crutches for 6 weeks. The average length of hospitalization was 5 days.

The disease associations are shown in Table 5. Eleven of 16 patients had bilateral disease at last follow-up, including 5 to 6 with alcohol-association INFH, 5 of 8 with steroid association, and the one patient with sickle cell disease. Six of these patients presented with bilateral disease at the time of initial consultation, while the other five developed symptoms in the second side while under follow-up for the more advanced side. In these five, all had had elevated BMP at the time of initial presentation for the first side. The second side had become symptomatic 2–8 months following the initial abnormal BMP.

Twenty-three patients with 23 hips underwent a core decompression for stage II disease. Results are shown in Table 4. Although seven had progressed to collapse, only four have needed further surgery. One of these has had a recoring procedure with a successfull follow-up of $2\frac{1}{2}$ years, and the other three have had total hip arthroplasties. The remaining three patients have minimal symptoms in spite of the X-ray progression. The disease-related associations are shown in Table 5. Of the 20 patients with nontraumatic INFH, 15 had developed bilateral disease at the time of the last follow-up. Eight patients originally presented with unilateral disease, of whom all but one had BMP measurement and stress test carried out on the initially asymptomatic radiologically negative side. The

Table 5. Disease association in stage I and stage II INFH

	Stage I	Stage II
Alcohol	8	6
Steroid	8	12
Trauma		3
Sickle cell	1	1
Idiopathic	1	1

three patients who subsequently developed INFH had abnormal BMP at the time of presentation for the contralateral side. Of the remaining patients, two had normal BMP and two had abnormal pressures, but they have not subsequently developed INFH. In one patient the test was not done.

Discussion

Even though the clinical X-ray examination remains the single most important tool in the diagnosis of INFH, reliance on the standard X-ray alone has led patients with stage I disease to be considered as not having bone necrosis. Even the subtle changes of stage II may be overlooked or considered nonspecific. The X-ray study becomes positive only after the circulatory changes have been either sufficiently extensive or prolonged to cause a change in the inorganic phase of bone. We have demonstrated that extensive marrow changes may be radiologically "silent". There are two important points concerning the usefulness of diagnostic X-ray. Although the earliest X-ray changes initially show no particular predilection for a given anatomical area within the head, the more obvious radiologic changes predominantly involve the anterolateral segment. Secondly, although the X-ray examination is of limited value in making an early diagnosis, it is of considerable value in staging. Once any deformity in the subchondral plate or early collapse of the supporting cancellous structure is radiologically evident, the prognosis is poor (Ficat et al. 1971; Hungerford and Zizic 1978; Marcus et al. 1973; Merle d'Aubigné et al. 1965).

Bone and bone marrow scanning with radionuclides are of great value if the X-ray study is negative and also in those patients with a high index of suspicion of INFH. Bone scanning is unnecessary if the X-ray is positive. Unfortunately, most patients have X-ray changes in at least one hip at the time when they are first seen by a physician. This represents a significant problem since the most sensitive reading of bone or bone marrow scans is on the basis of asymmetry. Inevitably, the more advanced side shows increased uptake on bone scan and decreased uptake on bone marrow scan. This means that for the second side the bone scan is of more limited usefulness. Only ten patients in this series had normal X-ray studies and a unilaterally symptomatic hip. Of these, seven had positive bone scans characterized by increased uptake on the symptomatic side. The remaining three were interpreted as normal. However, the contralateral side became symptomatic within a few weeks or months of the first side, so that in retrospect, there was probably mild bilaterally symmetrical increase in uptake. It is hoped that computerized quantitative scintigraphy will make it possible, in the future, to evaluate a single hip without the need for a normal opposite side for comparison. In our experience with patients with SLE and bone necrosis, 14 of 27 sides were falsely interpreted as negative (Zizic et al. 1980). In each case the site had been either confirmed histologically or showed the typical X-ray changes. Thirteen of the 14 false negative sites were in patients with bilateral involvement. Thus, although the uptake was read as normal, it is possible that it could have been increased, but to a lesser extent than the more severely affected side.

Bone marrow pressure elevation strongly correlates with INFH in all stages and is particularly useful in stages I and II where the X-ray is of little value and where the bone scan may be compromised by more advanced disease on the opposite side. It also appears to be of use in designating the hip at risk in patients with unilateral disease, since we have found a high correlation between elevated BMP and the subsequent development of INFH. These patients can then be followed up more closely in order to intercept that hip in the earliest symptomatic stages of the disease rather than after collapse has already occurred. To date we have not prophylactically carried out core decompression in any asymptomatic hips.

The exact role of elevated BMP in INFH and in other conditions affecting bone, both in terms of pathogenesis and production of symptoms, remains under some dispute. Several authors have recorded elevated BMP in osteoarthrosis of both the hips and knees (Arnoldi et al. 1972, 1975; Lynch 1974). Lynch (1974) correlated the degree of pain with the degree of proximal tibial intraosseous hypertension in patients presenting for high tibial osteotomy and unicompartmental osteoarthrosis of the knee. However, in osteoarthrosis as contrasted to INFH, the degree of the roentgenographic abnormality correlates directly to the degree of intraosseous hypertension and venographic abnormalities (Arnoldi et al. 1972; Lynch 1974). The BMP findings in osteoarthrosis are presumably secondary to the remodeling and trabecular hypertrophy, which is due to the abnormal joint-loading associated with cartilage loss. The findings in INFH suggest strongly that the BMP changes play a more important pathogenetic role in the evolution of the condition. This is particularly strengthened by the finding of increased BMP in the asymptomatic and radiologically normal contralateral hip of patients with unilateral disease who then go on to develop symptoms and X-ray changes of the second side.

Pathogenesis

The concepts of pathogenesis and etiology must be separated. It is obvious from the disease-related conditions that there are multiple etiological associations with nontraumatic INFH. And yet the clinical and radiological presentation and evolution are remarkably similar. There are basically two broad pathogenetic concepts which have been widely reported. The first concept is that the bone in the anterolateral segment infarcts rather quickly. This could come about either by occlusion of the posterolateral retinacular vessel or by emboli from a variety of sources finding their way into the microcirculation in the subchondral region of bone. The subsequent collapse would then be on the basis of revascularization of the necrotic segment (Glimcher and Kenzora 1979). This would weaken the trabecular structure, resulting in the accumulation of microfractures and collapse of the weight-bearing segment of the femoral head. This concept fits both the typical radiologic appearance and the histologic findings in femoral heads removed at the time of replacement. The histologic support for this concept comes, however, from the advanced stages of the disease. There can be little doubt that, once the collapse starts, there is indeed an infarcted segment involving primarily the anterolateral segment of the femoral head. The question to be resolved, however, is whether or not this segment has been infarcted from the very earliest stages of the disease.

The second pathogenetic concept is that the bone functions as a closed compartment and that the eventual infarction of the weight-bearing bone is the end stage of a slowly progressive compartment syndrome (Hungerford 1979). The finding of elevated BMP in all stages of INFH, and even in a preclinical stage, supports this concept. As the bone becomes progressively ischemic, the greatest effect is experienced in the weight-bearing area, where microfractures are not repaired and consequently accumulate, and the collapse proceeds. The end stages of the two concepts are virtually superimposable. The starting points are at opposite ends of the spectrum.

Wilkes and Visscher (1975) have shown that bone does indeed function under normal circumstances as a closed compartment. Changes in BMP must result in inversely proportional changes in bone blood flow, unless there is an increase in the pressure of flow which is delivered to the bone. There are no indications that bone has any independent autoregulatory mechanisms. In fact, any process which evokes bone ischemia is likely to result in increased BMP, which would then potentiate the ischemia. By this mechanism such possible divergent etiologies as steroid- or alcohol-induced fat embolism (Jones 1971) to bone as well as the intraosseous lipocyte hypertrophy mechanism of Wang et al. (1977) could produce the similar effects of increased BMP and decreased bone blood flow.

It is even possible that posttraumatic INFH may evolve through a similar mechanism. Although it cannot be questioned that bone may be infarcted following fracture of the femoral neck or dislocation of the hip, it is certainly possible that a lesser degree of ischemia, which was begun at the time of the injury, could proceed along the mechanism of increased BMP and progressive ischemia, eventually resulting in bone death. Jacqueline and Rabinowitz (1973), in studying the histology of 62 femoral heads from several days to many months after fracture of the femoral neck, concluded that there was no

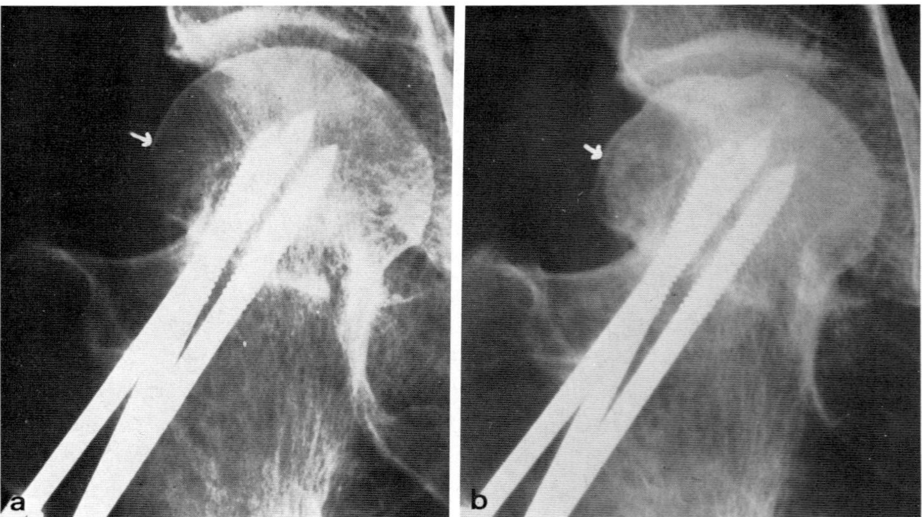

Fig. 11a, b. A young patient with an impacted valgus fracture of the femoral neck. The *arrow* marks the original lateral margin of contact of the acetabulum with the femoral head before the fracture. **a** Six months after the injury, the fracture has healed and the patient is asymptomatic. **b** Fifteen months after the fracture, the *new* weight-bearing area is collapsing (Hungerford 1979)

evidence of sudden and extensive necrosis after fracture, but rather a slowly progressive necrosis in both extent and depth. Those patients who had resumed walking showed the most extensive lesions in the weight-bearing areas. One of our patients who sustained an impacted valgus fracture of the femoral neck showed progressive change in the new weight-bearing area rather than in the anatomical anterolateral segment (Fig. 11).

This second pathogenetic concept, to which we subscribe, suggests that ischemia provokes bone marrow edema and fibrosis which elevates BMP. This results in a further decrease in bone blood flow, potentiating the ischemia. The cycle of ischemia, edema, and increased pressure culminates in bone death. The mechanical failure and eventual collapse results from weight-bearing being superimposed on ischemic bone. The work of Wang et al. (1977), demonstrating increased intramedullary lipocyte size associated with increased BMP in rabbits treated with steroids, and the work of Pooley and Walder (1980), demonstrating increased lipocyte size in animals treated with compressed air and a concomittant decrease in bone blood flow, suggest that bone marrow pressure changes may be primary in the production of the ischemia as well.

Treatment

Once there are changes evident in the X-ray examination, medical management, consisting of protective weight-bearing, analgesics, and anti-inflammatory agents, has been shown to be ineffective (Romer and Wettstein 1971). No control studies employing prolonged protective weight-bearing in the preradiologic stage of the disease have appeared. Taking a biopsy to confirm the diagnosis, without which the diagnosis must be presumptive, provides treatment both in decompressing the bone and in stimulation vascular neogenesis. Therefore, the result of medical management in the preradiologic stage of INFH is unknown.

Core biopsy offers the opportunity to study the earliest changes of bone ischemia histologically. It also provides a rapid decrease in symptoms and in the precollapse stages is associated with a low incidence of progressive changes in the femoral head. Even though the presence of BMP elevation has lead to a high incidence of the development of symptomatic INFH, elevated BMP alone has not been universally associated with progressive disease. From our results and those reported by Ficat and Arlet (1980), we believe core decompression to be the procedure of choice in the preradiologic and precollapse stages of INFH.

Other procedures have been suggested as means of preserving the femoral head in more advanced stages of the disease. Several authors have reported the partial success of musculopedicle graft (Phemister 1949), tibial or fibular grafts (Boettcher et al. 1970; Bonfiglio and Voke 1968; Marcus et al. 1975; Phemister 1949), repositioning osteotomies (Kerboul et al. 1974; Merle d'Aubigne et al. 1965; Wagner 1964; Wang et al. 1980), and free vascularized bone grafts. In each case the results were proportional to the degree of head involvement and the extent of radiologic change. It would appear that early diagnosis is the key to success of all preservative methods of treatment of INFH. A high index of suspicion in those patients falling into the susceptible disease categories and the utilization of the diagnostic measures which are currently available should lead to earlier diagnosis and better treatment results for patients with INFH.

References

Arlet J, Ficat P (1968) Diagnostic de l'ostéonécrose fémoro-capitale au stade I. Rev Chir Orthop 54:637

Arnoldi CC, Linderholm H, Mussbichler H (1972) Venous engorgement and intraosseous hypertension in osteoarthritis of the hip. J Bone Joint Surg [Br] 54:409

Arnoldi CC, Lemperg RK, Linderholm H (1975) Intraosseous hypertension and pain in the knee. J Bone Joint Surg [Br] 3:360

Boettcher WG, Bonfiglio M, Smith K (1970) Non-traumatic necrosis of the femoral head. Part II. Experiences in treatment. J Bone Joint Surg [Am] 52:322

Bonfiglio M, Voke EM (1968) Aseptic necrosis of the femoral head and non-union of the femoral head. J Bone Joint Surg [Am] 50:48

Chandler FA (1948) Coronary disease of the hip. J Int Coll Surg 11:34

Chung SMK, Ralston EL (1969) Necrosis of the femoral head associated with sickle-cell anemia and its genetic variants: a review of the literature and study of thirteen cases. J Bone Joint Surg [Am] 51:33

Cruess RL, Blennerhassett J, Macdonald FR, MacLean LD, Dossetor J (1968) Aseptic necrosis following renal transplantation. J Bone Joint Surg [Am] 50:1577

Dubois EL (1960) Avascular (aseptic) bone necrosis associated with systemic lupus erythematosus. JAMA 174:966

Edstrom G (1961) Destruction of hip-joint in rheumatoid arthritis during long-term steroid therapy. Acta Rheum Scand 7:151

Ficat P, Arlet J (1968) Diagnostic de l'ostéonécrose fémoro-capitale primitive au stade I (stade préradiologique). Rev Chir Orthop 54:637

Ficat RP, Arlet J (1980) Ischemia and necroses of bone. Williams & Wilkins, Baltimore

Ficat P, et al. (1971) Resultats thérapeutiques du forage biopsie dans les ostéonécroses fémorocapitales primitives (100 cas). Rev Rhum Mal Osteoartic 38:269

Glimcher MJ, Kenzora JE (1979) The biology of osteonecrosis of the human femoral head and its clinical implications III. Clin Orthop 140:273

Harrington KD, Murray WR, Kountz SL, Belzer FO (1971) Avascular necrosis of bone after renal transplantation. J Bone Joint Surg [Am] 53:203

Hungerford DS (1975) Early diagnosis of ischemic necrosis of the femoral head. Johns Hopkins Med J 137:270

Hungerford DS (1979) Bone marrow pressure, venography, and core decompression in ischemic necrosis of the femoral head. In: The Hip. Proc. 1th Hip Soc. Meeting Mosby, St. Louis, p 218

Hungerford DS, Zizic TM (1972) Alcohol associated ischemic necrosis of the femoral head. Clin Orthop 130:144

Jacqueline F, Rabinowicz TH (1973) Lesions de la hanche secondaires à la fracture du col du fémur. In: Proceedings of the first international symposium on circulation of bone. Inserm, Paris, p 283

Jones JP (1971) Alcoholism, hypercortisonism, fat embolism and osseous avascular necrosis. In: Zinn WM (ed) Idiopathic ischemic necrosis of the femoral head in adults. Thieme, Stuttgart, p 112

Kerboul M, Thomine J, Postel M, Merle D'Aubigne R (1974) The conservative surgical treatment of idiopathic aseptic necrosis of the femoral head. J Bone Joint Surg [Br] 56:291

Larsen RM (1938) Intramedullary pressure with particular reference to massive diaphyseal bone necrosis: experimental observations. Ann Surg 108:127

Lynch JA (1974) Venous abnormalities and intraosseous hypertension associated with osteoarthritis of the knee. In: Ingweren O, et al. (eds) The knee joint. Excerpta Medica, Amsterdam, p 87

Mankin H, Brower TD (1962) Bilateral idiopathic aseptic necrosis of the femur in adults: Chandler's disease. Bull Hosp Joint Dis 23:42

Marcus ND, Enneking WF, Massam RA (1973) The silent hip in idiopathic aseptic necrosis. J Bone Joint Surg [Am] 55:1351

Merle D'Aubigne R, Postel M, Mazabraud A, et al. (1965) Idiopathic necrosis of the femoral head in adults. J Bone Joint Surg [Br] 47:612

Meyers MH (1978) The treatment of osteonecrosis of the hip with fresh osteochondral allografts and with the muscle pedicle graft technique. Clin Orthop 130:202

Phemister DB (1949) Treatment of the necrotic head of the femur in adults. J Bone Joint Surg [Am] 31:55

Pooley J, Walder DN (1980) Reduction in bone marrow blood flow during simulated dives: investigation of the mechanism. J Bone Joint Surg [Br] 62:635

Romer U, Wettstein P (1971) Results of treatment of eighty-one Swiss patients with INFH. In: Zinn WM (ed) Idiopathic ischemic necrosis of the femoral head in adults. University Park Press, Baltimore, p 205

Rutishauser E, Rhoner A, Held D (1960) Experimentelle Untersuchungen über die Wirkung der Ischämie auf den Knochen und das Mark. Virchows Arch [Pathol Anat] 33:101

Serre H, Simon L (1961) L'ostéonécrose primitive de la tête fémorale chez l'adulte. Acta Rheum Scand 7:265

Soloman L (1973) Drug-induced arthropathy and necrosis of the femoral head. J Bone Joint Surg [Br] 53:246

Sugioka K (1978) Transtrochanteric anterior rotational osteotomy of the femoral head in the treatment of osteonecrosis affecting the hip. Clin Orthop 130:191

Wagner H (1964) Behandlung der partiellen Hüftkopfnekrose. Verh Dtsch Orthop Ges [Suppl 51] 100:359

Wang GJ, Sweet DE, Reger SI, Thompson RC (1977) Fat cell changes as a mechanism of avascular necrosis of the femoral head in cortisone-treated rabbits. J Bone Joint Surg [Am] 59:729

Wang GJ, Lennox DW, Reger SI, Stamp RC, Hubbard S (1980) Cortisone induced intrafemoral head pressure changes and its response to drilling decompression method. Proc 26th Annu Orthop Res Soc 5:45

Wilkes CH, Visscher MB (1975) Some physiological aspects of bone marrow pressure. J Bone Joint Surg [Am] 57:49

Zizic TM, Hungerford DS, Stevens MB (1980) Ischemic necrosis of bone in systemic lupus erythematosus. I. Early diagnosis. Medicine (Baltimore) 59:134

Revitalization of the Osteonecrotic Femoral Head by Vascular Bundle Transplantation

Y. Hori

Great difficulty is met in the treatment of necrosis of the femoral head and other such bone diseases which are caused by avascular or hypovascular changes. It would seem logical to reconstruct a new vascular system for such lesions. With this in mind, vascular transplantation to bone was tried and investigated for subsequent changes of bone tissues and blood vessels (Hori et al. 1973, 1978, 1979).

In canine experiments, an artery, a vein, or a vascular bundle containing an artery and vein were transplanted into intact bones, isolated bones, necrotized bones, homografted bones, and necrotized femoral heads. It was verified that a vascular bundle which contained an artery and a vein produced microcirculation. Therefore, it was possible to revitalize an osteonecrotic femoral head by vascular bundle transplantation (Fig. 1). Based on the results of the experiment, vascular bundle transplantation has been applied in clinical cases, i.e., 40 cases (50 bones) of avascular necrosis of the femoral head, 11 of Perthes' disease, 17 of Kienboeck's disease, 5 of avascular necrosis of the scaphoid, 2 of avascular necrosis of the talus, and 2 in bone grafts for giant cell tumor of the tibia and nonunion of the humerus.

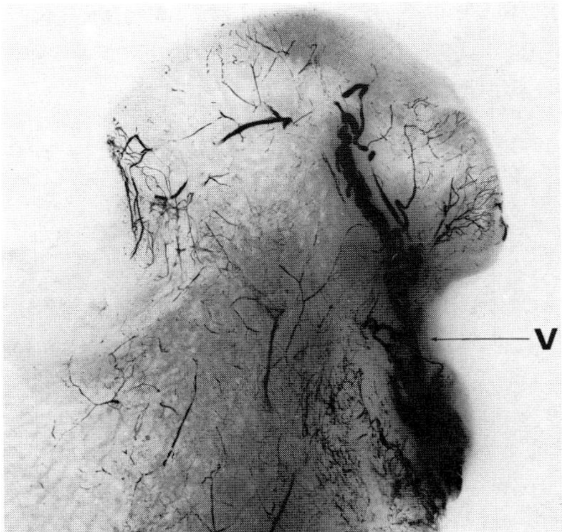

Fig. 1. Microangiogram of the femoral head, showing good revascularization 3 months after transplantation (*V*, transplanted vascular bundle)

In this paper, the vascular bundle transplantation for the avascular necrosis of the femoral head is described.

Operative Procedure

New instruments were made for this operation (Figs. 2, 3). The straight ventral incision, approximately 15 cm in length, begins cranial to the anterior superior iliac spine. The superficial and deep fascia is cut, and the proximal fourth of the sartorius and rectus femoris muscle is exposed. The sartorius muscle is retracted medially, and the rectus femoris muscle is divided from its origin and turned downward. The ascending branches of the lateral femoral circumflex artery and vein are isolated atraumatically as a single vascular bundle. Care must be taken not to sever either the artery or the vein. The transverse branches are isolated in the same way. The distal ends of these branches are ligated; a T-shaped incision is made in the capsule of the hip joint, and the femoral head is exposed.

A Kirschner wire is advanced from the subcapital region to the subchondral layer of the femoral head using an image amplifier. A cannulated reamer 6 mm in diameter is inserted over the Kirschner wire, and a hole is made. Necrotic tissue is curetted through the hole, and the cavity is filled with a cancellous bone graft. After this the reamed channel is cleaned of any remaining debris by reinserting the reamer. A cortical bone disk 6 mm in diameter is removed from the iliac bone by using a plug cutter and fixed to the end of the vascular bundle as an "anchor." The round cortical bone "anchor" is fixed on a special holding device, carried into the hole, and pushed through the channel. The bone anchor is fixed with a Kirschner wire during removal of the holding device. The iliopsoas musle is indented if the transplanted vascular bundle is compressed by it. This completes the vascular bundle transplantation. Postoperatively the patient remains in bed for 3 weeks with skin traction to the leg. Ambulation with crutches is then allowed for a minimum of 3 months. Ambulation without weight-bearing should be continued for a longer period in patients with advanced necrosis and severe deformity of the femoral head. Weight-bearing should be allowed gradually in all cases.

Case Reports

Case 1. A 53-year-old female after right femoral neck fracture and treated with a Smith-Peterson nail 5 years ago. X-ray examination 2 years after the operation revealed cyst formation in the femoral head. Observation over 6 months showed no sign of recovery but an increase of necrotic changes (Fig. 4a). The vascular bundle transplantation was performed 3 years after the injury. It was noted during surgery that the surface of the femoral head was dark yellow and that there was moderate deformity in the lateral part of the femoral head. A vascular bundle transplantation without bone graft was performed. The patient remained in bed for 3 weeks after operation, and ambulation with crutches was then allowed for 3 months. The cysts in the femoral head had almost disappeared 6

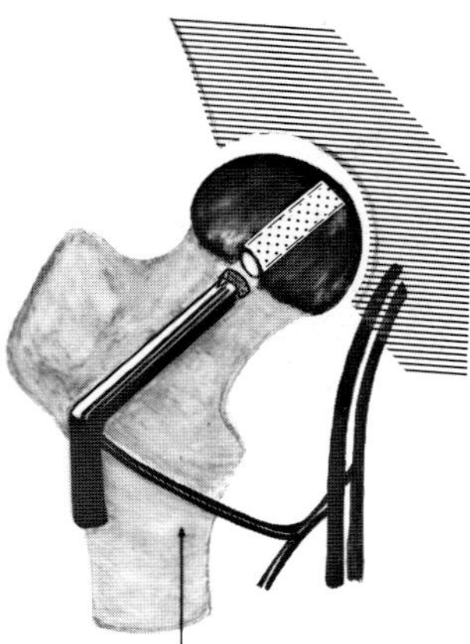

Fig. 2. Schema of vascular bundle transplantation for the femoral head

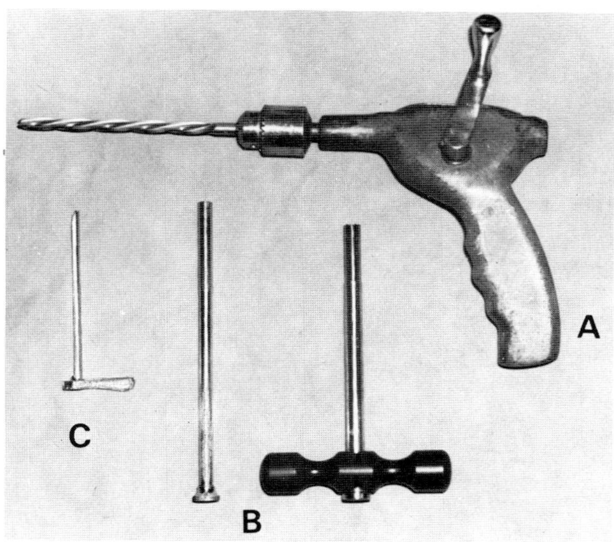

Fig. 3. Instruments for the transplantation. *A* reamer; *B* plug cutter; *C* holding device

months after the operation (Fig. 4b). Range of motion of the hip joint became almost normal. The patient returned to her usual life as a housewife 6 months after the operation and had no complaints 3 years after the operation (Fig. 4c). The bone scan became almost normal.

Case 2. A 17-year-old boy with a history of right hip joint pain for 2 years prior to his first visit. The motion of his right hip joint was limited (flexion: 80°). Roentgenogram showed

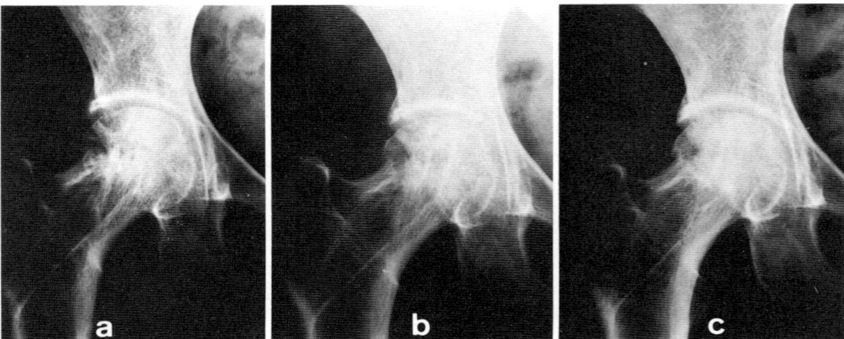

Fig. 4a–c. Roentgenogram of the femoral head of case 1. **a** preoperative view, showing cyst formation; **b** 6 months after the transplantation; **c** 3 years after the transplantation, showing that cysts in the femoral head have disappeared

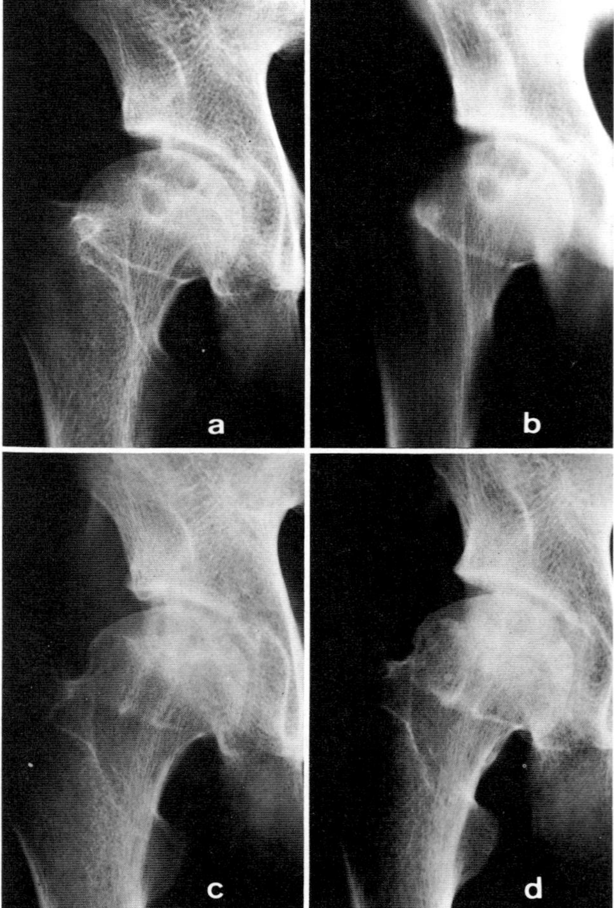

Fig. 5a–d. Roentgenogram of the femoral head of case 2. **a** preoperative view showing extensive cyst formation in the femoral head; **b** preoperative tomogram; **c** 3 months after the transplantation; **d** 18 months after the transplantation showing that cystic changes have disappeared

cyst formation in the femoral head (Fig. 5a, b). Intraoperatively a hypertrophic articular capsule and yellowish articular cartilage were noted. After curettage of necrotic tissue, the vascular bundle transplantation with a cancellous bone graft was performed. The patient remained in bed for 4 weeks, then ambulation with crutches was allowed. Cysts in the femoral head had almost disappeared 3 months after surgery (Fig. 5c). The patient returned to his normal life as a student 6 months after surgery. The X-ray examination 18 months after surgery revealed that cystic shadows had disappeared and that the femoral head was restored (Fig. 5d). The range of motion of the hip joint was almost normal, and clinical symptoms were absent.

Case 3. A 39-year-old male who was suffering from rheumatoid arthritis and had been treated with steroids. Five years ago, avascular necrosis was detected in his left femoral head, and an intertrochanteric valgus osteotomy was performed in the left femur (Fig. 6a). Two years ago, 3 years after the osteotomy, he complained of severe pain in both hip joints, and was referred to us. X-ray examination revealed that the left femoral head was severely damaged and that there was an extensive infraction in the right femoral head (Fig. 6b). During the operation, yellowish articular cartilage and deformity of the femoral head was noted. After curettage of necrotic tissue, vascular bundle transplantation with cancellous bone graft was performed. After 3 weeks of bed rest, ambulation with crutches was allowed. The sclerotic area and the fracture line disappeared 6 months after surgery (Fig. 6c).

Figure 6d is a roentgenogram taken 18 months after surgery. The deformity of the femoral head was improved, and there were areas of proliferating bone around the drill hole which corresponded well with results of the animal experiment. Range of motion of the hip joint had increased, and pain had decreased.

Case 4. A 40-year-old male who had suffered from left hip joint pain for 1 year. Limitation of the hip joint was noted (flexion: 80°) during the first examination. X-ray examination revealed deformity and large cysts in the femoral head (Fig. 7a, b). Intraoperatively, a thickened articular capsule and folds of yellowish degenerative articular cartilage easily dented by digital pressure were noted. There were large cysts demarcated by sclerotic bone inside the femoral head.

After curettage of necrotic tissues, the vascular bundle transplantation with cancellous bone graft was performed. After 4 weeks of bed rest, ambulation with crutches was allowed. Two months after surgery, the cysts in the femoral head had almost disappeared (Fig. 7c). Ten months after surgery, the patient returned to his life as a laborer. Cystic changes had disappeared 1 year after surgery in the roentgenogram, and the patient had no clinical symptoms (Fig. 7d).

Discussion

Since Vinberg's (1946) report on successful vascular transplantation into the cardiac muscle, similar studies have been conducted by many others. Woodhouse (1963) reported on transplantation of the brachial artery into the humerus using dogs, describing that arterial anastomosis occurred between the transplanted artery and preexisting arteries. Dickerson and Duthie transplanted the femoral artery of a dog into the femur and noted

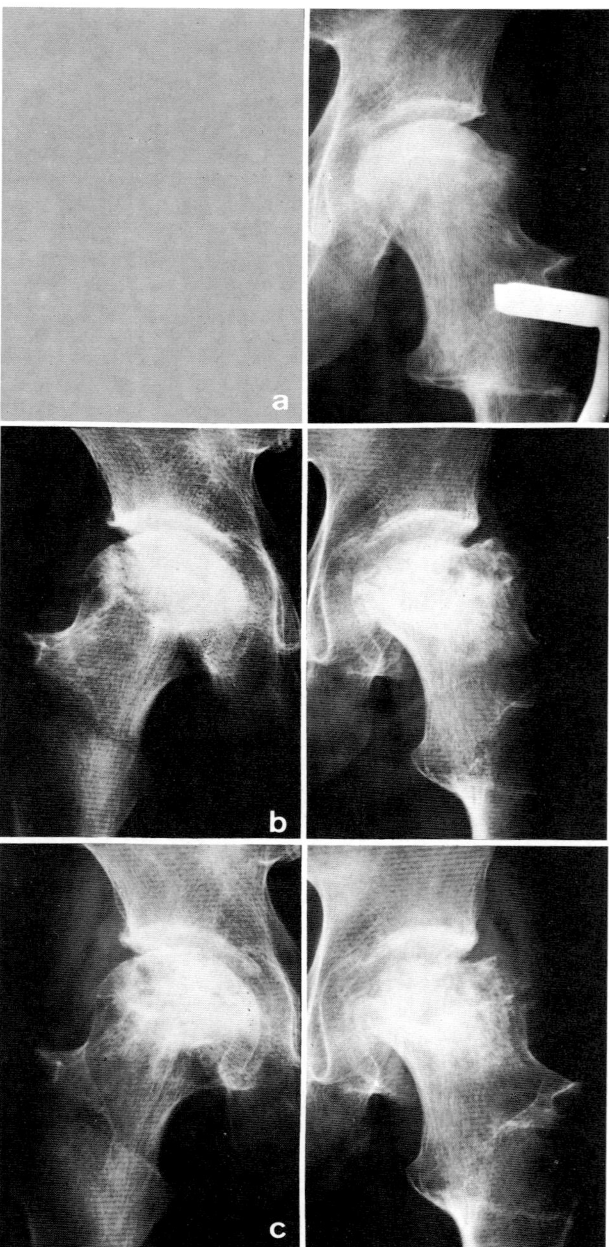

Fig. 6a–d. Roentgenogram of the femoral head of case 3. **a** Left, femoral head 3 months after osteotomy. **b** *Right*, preoperative view, showing sclerosis, deformity, and infraction in the femoral head.
Left, 3 years after the osteotomy. **c** *Right,* 6 months after the transplantation, showing that fracture
line disappeared. The left hip is unchanged. **d** *Right*, 18 months after the transplantation, showing
that deformity of the femoral head was restored and that there is proliferating bone around the drill
hole

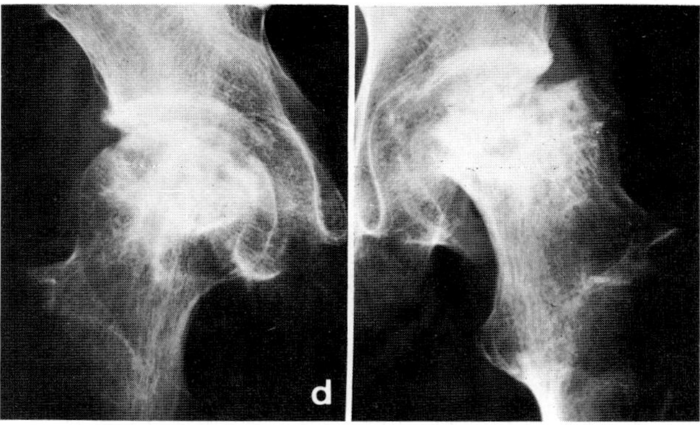

Fig. 6d

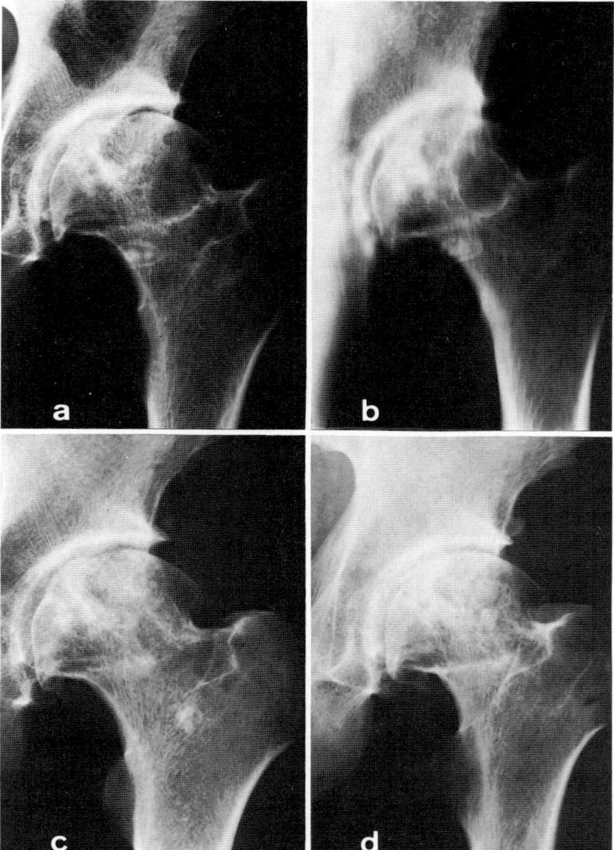

Fig. 7a–d. Roentgenogram of the femoral head of case 4. **a** preoperative view showing concave deformity and cysts in the femoral head; **b** preoperative tomogram; **c** 2 months after the transplantation; **d** 1 year after transplantation; cystic changes have disappeared

proliferation of blood vessels and new bone (Dickerson and Duthie 1963; Dickerson 1966, 1968). Boyd and Ault (1965) transplanted the femoral artery into the femoral neck in dogs and found the transplanted artery to be patent. The method used by Dickerson and Boyd is different from ours; they used tubes to infuse the blood into the bone marrow cavity and transplanted only an *artery* into intact bone.

Our experiments verified that a transplanted artery into an isolated bone soon became occluded, which seemed to be caused by a lack of efferent blood flow. Arterial transplantation alone cannot revitalize necrotic bone. The experiments also verified that, with the vascular bundle transplantation containing an artery and a vein, revascularization occurred in isolated bone, necrotized bone, and in 66% of the homografts. They also confirmed that necrotized femoral heads, which were caused experimentally by interruption of blood supply, could be fully revitalized by the vascular bundle transplantation. On the basis of the experimental results, vascular bundle transplantation has been suitable for clinical cases. The longest follow-up term is 5 years, and results are satisfactory.

Vascular bundle transplantation can revitalize a necrotic femoral head, but cannot completely restore severe deformities of the femoral head. It is well suited for early stages of femoral head necrosis. In cases of extensive advanced necrosis of the femoral head, vascular bundle transplantation combined with a spongiosa graft is indicated in an attempt to restore good remodeling of the femoral head. Long periods of postoperative non-weight-bearing are required in such cases. Secondary operations to improve congruency, i.e., femoral osteotomy, may be necessary if arthrotic changes develop at a later date.

Summary

The procedure of my original method for the treatment of avascular necrosis, vascular bundle transplantation, has been described, and clinical cases were presented.

References

Boyd RJ, Ault LL (1965) An experimental study of vascular implantation into the femoral head. Surg Gynecol Obstet 121:1009

Dickerson RC (1966) The diversion of arterial blood flow to growing bone. Surg Gynecol Obstet 123:103

Dickerson RC (1968) An improved method for diversion of arterial blood flow to bone. J Bone Joint Surg [Am] 50:1036

Dickerson RC, Duthie RB (1963) The division of arterial blood flow to bone. J Bone Joint Surg [Am] 45:356

Hori Y, et al. (1973) Blood vessel transplantation to bone, the first report. J Jpn Orthop Assoc 47:252

Hori Y, et al. (1978) Blood vessel transplantation to bone. J Jpn Orthop Assoc 52:25

Hori Y, et al. (1979) Blood vessel transplantation to bone. J Hand Surg 4:23

Vineberg AM (1946) Development of an anastomosis between the coronary vessels and transplanted internal mammary artery. Can Med Assoc J 55:117

Woodhouse CF (1963) The transplantation of patent arteries to bone. J Int Coll Surg 39:437

Translation from the German: Hori Y (1980) Revitalisierung des osteonekrotischen Hüftkopfes durch Gefäßbündel-Transplantation. Orthopädie 9:255–259 © Springer Verlag 1980

Transstrochanteric Ventral Rotation Osteotomy After Sugioka for Treatment of Femoral Head Necrosis

R. Kotz

Introduction

Various operation methods can change the position of the femoral head. These are varization, valgization, flexion, and rotational osteotomies (Cartier et al. 1972; Endler 1972; Merle d'Aubigné et al. 1965; Sugioka 1973; Willert and Sarfer 1974). With Sugioka's method for avascular necrosis of the femoral head, a maximum of correction of the joint surface can be obtained (Fig. 1).

Because of poor results with joint-preserving operative methods at the Department of Orthopedic Surgery at the University of Vienna from 1965 to 1975, Sugioka's method was adopted for avascular necrosis of the hip joint in 1975. Twenty-four cases were operated on in the last 4 years, using the transtrochanteric ventral rotational osteotomy. The results have been clinically evaluated after an observation period of 5–48 months (mean 22.5 months) and were compared with the results of the joint-preserving operations from 1965 to 1975.

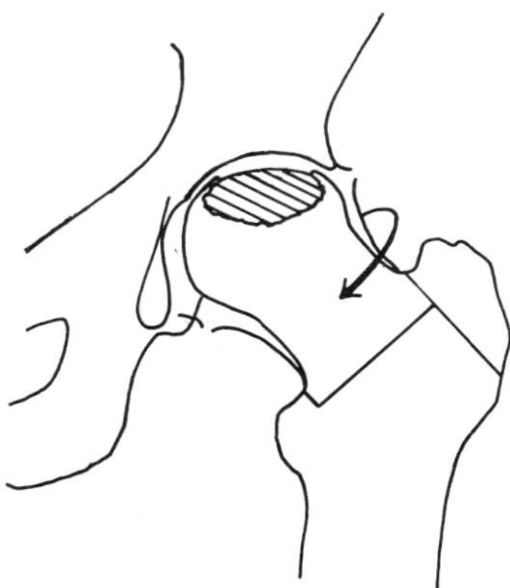

Fig. 1. Transtrochanteric anterior rotation osteotomy ("Sugioka") with incision of the capsule near the acetabulum (Sugioka 1973, 1978, 1980)

Case Material

Twenty-four patients with avascular femoral head necrosis were selected for the operation (22 males and 2 females, 17–57 years old, with an average age of 37.5 years) (Table 1). The prerequisites were full extension of the hip with a minimum flexion of 90° and an intact posterior joint space demonstrated by Schneider's roentgenogram technique (Schneider 1970) (Fig. 2). All cases showed necroses of the femoral head with a necrotic conical angle of 85°–120°, mean values being 100.4° (±14.1) (Kotz and Ramach 1978). The necrosis was always localized anterocranially (Fig. 3).

Table 1. Data concerning twenty-four patients with avascular necrosis of the femoral head

Sex	22 ♂ 2 ♀	
Age	17–57 years,	⌀ 37.7 (± 8.6)
Necrotic conical		
Angle	85°–120°,	⌀ 100.4° (± 14.1)

⌀ = average

Method

Transtrochanteric osteotomy perpendicular to the femoral neck is performed after removal of the greater trochanter and incision of the capsule near the acetabulum (Fig. 4). Anterior rotation should be 70°–90°. The osteotomy is fixed with screws. The first five cases were approached anterolaterally according to Watson-Jones and were immobilized in plaster spicas after operation. Twelve patients were operated on by using Sugioka's approach, but on a fracture table. The remaining seven cases were operated on in a lateral position according to Sugioka. The external rotators are exposed and transected. The a. capitis femoris lateralis is spared. In this way, it is possible to perform a ventral femoral head rotation of 80°–90° without endangering the blood supply of the femoral head. Osteosynthesis was accomplished by using 3–4 screws. The trochanter was reat-

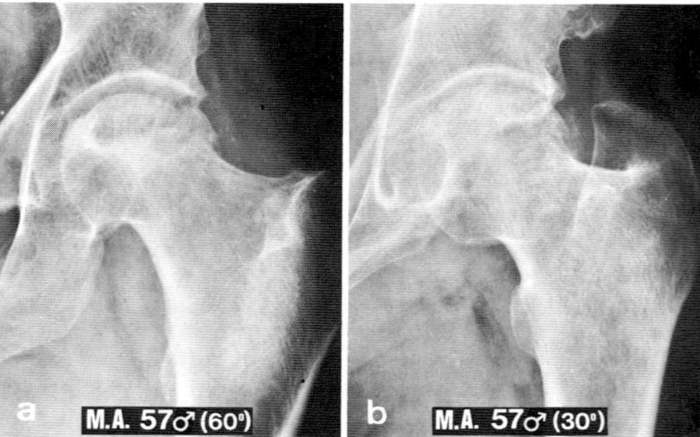

Fig. 2a, b. M.A., 57-year-old male patient with an avascular necrosis of the left hip. **a** Schneider's roentgenogram with 60° flexion of the hip joint. **b** The X-ray with inclination of the tubus 30° cranially shows the intact posterior joint space

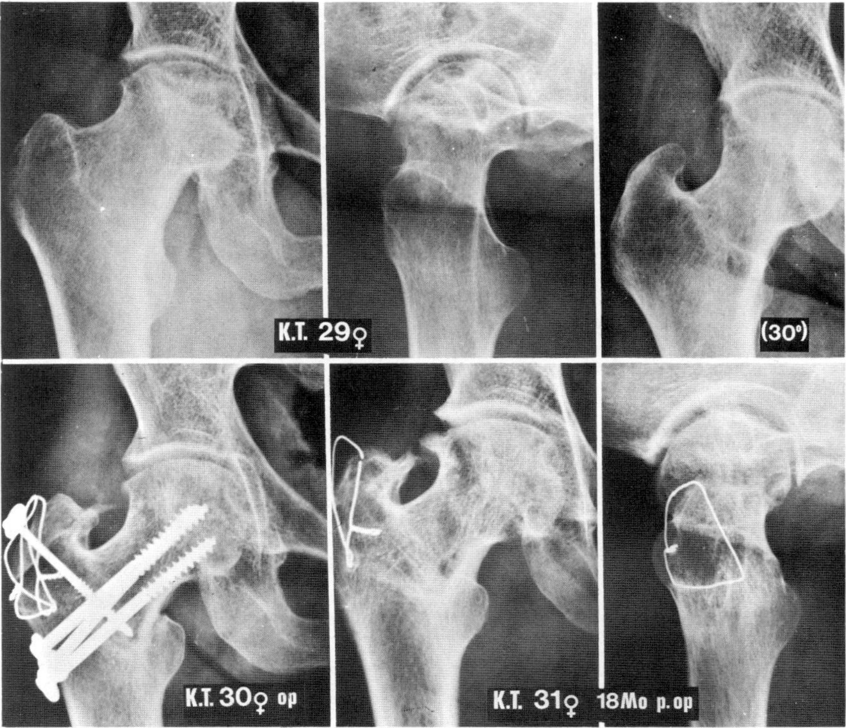

Fig. 3a–f. K.T., 29-year-old female patient with bilateral avascular necrosis of the hip, which had occurred during pregnancy. **a** Anterioposterior and **b** axial roentgenogram shows the anterocranial localization of the necrosis. **c** Schneider's roentgenogram shows the intact posterior joint space. **d** Sugioka's osteotomy on the right hip was performed post partum. **e, f** An excellent clinical result was obtained 18 months after operation

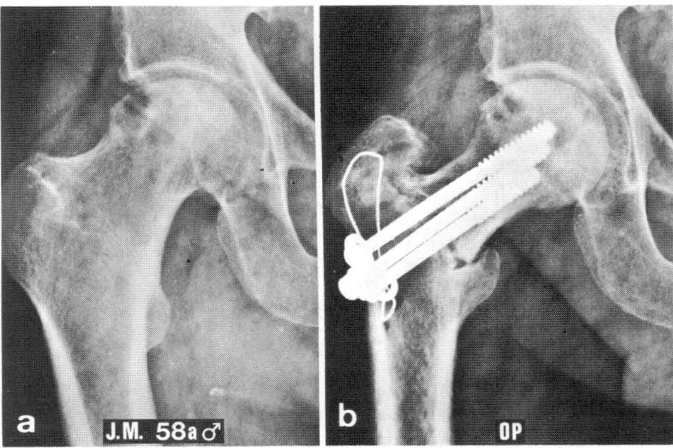

Fig. 4a, b. J.M., 58-year-old male patient. **a** Idiopathic avascular necrosis of the right hip. **b** A ventral rotation of 90° was done, the weight-bearing surface could be replaced by an intact part of the femoral head

tached either with screws or with wire cerelage. In two cases the trochanter was not fixed
in order to obtain muscle relaxation. The angle of ventral rotation was 45°–90°, mean
value was 67.5° (±15.3) (Table 2).

Table 2. Angles of anterior rotation and grades of necrosis in the previously mentioned twenty-four
patients with avascular necrosis of the femoral head

Angle of anterior rotation			
40–90°,	⌀ 67.5°	(± 14.1)	n = 24
Grade of necrosis			
I (n = 3),	II (n = 20),	III (n = 1)	

⌀ = average

Postoperative Treatment

During the first postoperative week, the hip is kept in 30° flexion. Skin traction of 2 kg is
employed. In cases of a marked external rotation tendency, internal rotation traction of
1–2 kg is applied. During the first postoperative week the joint is *slowly* extended. The
reason for this is to avoid sudden compression of the bone-supplying artery, which is
stretched by ventral rotation. Passive exercises are performed during the second and
third postoperative weeks, and active exercises are carried out during the 4th week. The
patient begins to ambulate without weight-bearing on the operated limb on the 28th day
after surgery. Partial weight-bearing on the operated hip is permitted 3 months after surgery, and the Lofstrand crutches are gradually discarded during the 4th–6th postoperative month.

Clinical Evaluation

The postoperative time of observation was 5–48 months, with a mean of 22.5 (±11.8
months). Clinical results were judged according to Patterson's scheme (Table 3). Seven
patients had an excellent result, nine patients had a good result, and five patients had
improved, including four patients with a necrotic conical angle of 120° (Table 4). One
patient required an arthroplasty 3.5 years after the rotation osteotomy because of progressive joint deterioration. Two patients with postoperative complications had a very poor
result. The best results were obtained in patients with osteonecrosis angles below 90°.

Complications

The angle between neck and shaft shifted 20°–30° into a varus position in five patients
during follow-up observation; one of them had to be revalgizised. The other patients
healed with a slight varus position, and compensated it well clinically. Another compli-

Table 3. Clinical results judged according to Patterson's scheme

Patient	Age	Sex	Extent of necrosis[a]	Angle of rotation	Months of observ.	Results[b]	Secondary treatment
H. M.	46	♀	110°	45°	48	+	Valg. Ost.
Sch. J.	35	♂	80°	60°	33	+++	−
R. W.	35	♂	120°	40°	31	+	−
F. J.	43	♂	90°	70°	43	++	−
S. J.	54	♂	90°	70°	26	++	Fracture, Nailing, Valg. Ost.
S. A.	32	♂	90°	70°	24	+++	−
K. T.	29	♀	90°	70°	22	+++	−
M. Ku.	47	♂	105°	50°	40	−	Endoprosthesis
M. Kl.	36	♂	120°	60°	21	−−	Total necrosis, endoprosthesis
Sch. A.	17	♂	95°	60°	12	−−	Arthrodesis (21) Rearthrodesis
L. F.	38	♂	120°	70°	20	+	−
V. A.	44	♂	85°	60°	34	+++	−
K. F.	28	♂	120°	60°	31	+	−
St. F.	33	♂	95°	60°	11	++	−
C. A.	39	♂	120°	45°	29	++	−
R. A.	36	♂	90°	60°	13	++	−
P. S.	45	♂	110°	60°	25	++	−
J. M.	57	♂	100°	90°	16	−−	−
E. A.	37	♂	90°	80°	12	++	−
R. G.	31	♂	120°	90°	50	+	−
K. K.	38	♂	110°	90°	13	+++	−
B. H.	39	♂	80°	80°	8	++	−
J. W.	36	♂	90°	90°	12	++	−
St. H.	29	♂	90°	90°	5	+	−

[a] Extent of necrosis: necrotic conical angle (Kotz and Ramach 1978)

[b] Results: +++, excellent; ++, good; +, improved; −, poor; −−, very poor (Patterson et al. 1964)

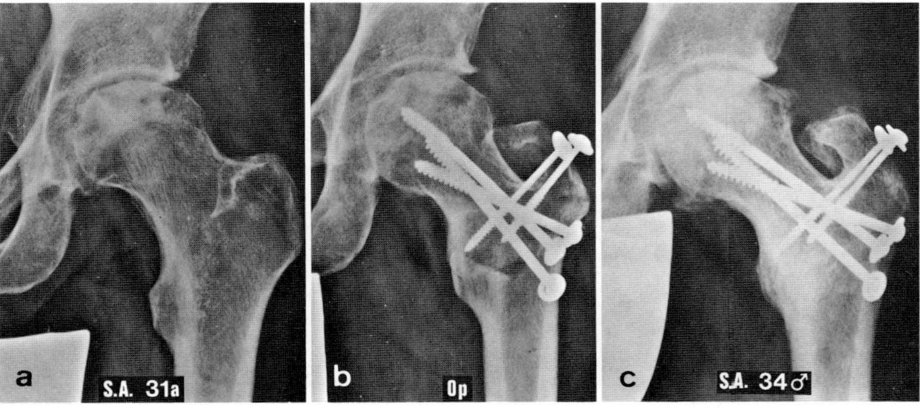

Fig. 5a–c. S.A., 31-year-old male patient. **a** Avascular necrosis of the left hip. **b** After ventral rotational osteotomy of 70°, the weight-bearing surface was restored. **c** The patient was without pain and could walk freely 23 months after operation. Though there are signs of osteoarthrosis in the X-ray, he can bear full weight

Table 4. Improvement in patients according to the necrotic conical angle

Necrotic conical angle	Results (Patterson et al. 1964)				
	Excellent	Good	Improved	Poor	Very poor
– 90°	5	6	–	–	–
95–115°	2	2	1	1	1
120°	–	1	4	–	1

cation was severe deep infection with osteomyelitis. In this case an arthrodesis, followed by rearthrodesis because of pseudarthrosis, had to be performed. In another case with an initially good postoperative result, the patient developed a complete necrosis of the femoral head 1 year later, and a total endoprosthesis had to be implanted. In another case, 6 months after Sugioka's osteotomy, a fracture of the femoral neck occurred after removal of the screws, and it had to be nailed. Because of a nail fracture, a 30° valgization and renailing had to be performed, and a satisfactory result was finally achieved. The other 17 patients were free of complications.

Discussion

Follow-up studies of intertrochanteric osteotomies and myotomies for femoral head necroses from 1965 to 1975 showed that grade III femoral head necroses with clear signs of arthrosis yielded poor results for joint-preserving operations (Kotz 1976). This experience influenced our decision to use Sugioka's osteotomy. Less importance was attributed to the relatively poor results of extensive femoral head necroses. Analysis of the operations showed that poor postoperative results increased parallel to the increase of the size of the necroses. When the necrosis angle was more than 120°, a joint-preserving method failed in most cases.

A comparison of the results of 24 Sugioka osteotomies having an average follow-up period of 22.5 months with the results of 25 intertrochanteric osteotomies and myotomies from 1965 to 1975 (follow-up observation: 1–10 years) definitely favors Sugioka's osteotomy (Table 5). But follow-up studies are not yet long enough to allow evaluation of

Table 5. Comparison of the results of 24 Sugioka osteotomies with 25 intertrochanteric osteotomies and myotomies

	Excellent	Good	Improved	Poor	Very poor	Better: Worse
Transtrochanteric anterior rotational osteotomy (1975–1978)	5	5	4	1	2	14 : 2
Intertrochanteric osteotomy and myotomy (1965–1975)	3	4	4	1	13	11 : 14

long-term results. The ratio good: poor in the Sugioka group is 21:3 versus 11:14 in the historic group. Even taking into account that five patients of the historic group had a grade III necrosis while only one patient treated with the Sugioka method belonged to this group, the results of the Sugioka group are still more favorable.

Conclusions

Due to the favorable results of Sugioka's transtrochanteric ventral rotational osteotomy, the indication for this joint-preserving operation in some cases of avascular femoral head necrosis is justified. Results were especially favorable in cases of early stages and in cases of small and medium-sized necroses. Problems arise for ventral rotational osteotomy when necroses exceed 120°. Moreover, rotational osteotomy should not be performed on grade III necroses with distinct signs of arthrosis. The technically difficult operation bears the risk of complications, necessitating secondary operations. Nevertheless results are favorable, even for patients with secondary operations, so that Sugioka's osteotomy should be considered in the therapy of avascular femoral head necrosis.

Addendum

Last year we changed our mobilization scheme. Patients were permitted to get out of bed 21 days postoperatively. The use of the Lofstrand crutches was reduced to 8–10 weeks. Of ten additional patients who underwent surgery last year and who were mobilized more quickly, four developed a pseudarthrosis because of late varization of the neck-shaft angle. Therefore, quicker mobilization increases complications and cannot be permitted.

References

Cartier O, Hautier S, Lemoire A (1972) L'ostéotomie de variation dans la nécrose idiopathique de la tête fémorale. Ann Chir 26:483

Endler F (1972) Traitement biomécanique chirurgical de la nécrose avasculaire de la tête fémorale. Acta Orthop Belg 38:537

Kotz R (1976) Die operative Therapie der idiopathischen Hüftkopfnekrose mit besonderer Berücksichtigung der Endoprothese. Orthop Prax 12:669

Kotz R, Pflüger G (1977) Die transtrochantäre ventrale Rotationsosteotomie bei der Behandlung der idiopathischen Hüftkopfnekrose. Acta Chir Austriaca 9:65

Kotz R, Ramach W (1978) Zur Bestimmung der Nekrosegröße durch ein Winkelmaß bei der idiopathischen Hüftkopfnekrose. Roentgenpraxis 31:1–7

Merle d'Aubigne R, Postel M, Mazabraud A, Massias P, Gueguen J (1965) Idiopathic necrosis of the femoral head in adults. J Bone Joint Surg [Br] 47:612

Patterson RJ, Bickel WB, Dahlin DC (1964) Idiopathic avascular necrosis of the head of the femur. J Bone Joint Surg [Am] 46:267

Sugioka Y (1973) Transtrochanteric anterior rotation osteotomy of the femoral head for avascular
    necrosis in adults. Cent Jpn J Orthop Traum Surg 16:574
Sugioka Y (1978) Transtrochanteric anterior rotational osteotomy of the femoral head in the
    treatment of osteonecrosis affecting the hip – a new osteotomy. Clin Orthop 130:191
Sugioka Y (1980) Transtrochanteric rotational osteotomy of the femoral head. The Hip: Proc.
    8th meet. Hip Soc.: 3
Willert HG, Sarfert D (1974) Die operative Behandlung der segmentalen Hüftnekrose. Z Orthop
    112:694

Translation from the German: Kotz R (1980) Die transtrochantere ventrale Rotationsosteotomie
nach Sugioka zur Behandlung der Femurkopfnekrose. Orthopäde 9:260–264 © Springer Verlag
1980

Results of Flexion Osteotomy on Segmental Femoral Head Necrosis in Adults

H.G. Willert, G. Buchhorn, L. Zichner

Since 1970, the syndrome of segmental femoral head necrosis (also called idiopathic, aseptic, or avascular femoral head necrosis) has been observed with increasing frequency. This is particularly important since, as a rule, young adults are affected, and as yet there is no method of treatment which can definitely cure the process once characteristic morphological changes have developed. Without treatment, segmental femoral head necrosis results in destruction of the joint: While the overlying articular cartilage remains vital, there is usually a demarcation zone between the necrotic segment and surrounding living bone due to a space filled with fibrous tissue, which can be compared to pseudarthrosis. With weight-bearing pressure, the necrotic segment collapses, resulting in progressive deformity of the femoral head. A characteristic arthrosis develops in reaction to this. Since segmental femoral head necrosis in itself rarely causes discomfort (Willert 1977), it is not noticed in many cases until deformity of the femoral head has already occurred.

Diagnostic Radiology

Necrosis generally affects a cranioventral segment of the femoral head. The spongiosa of the dorsal section of the femoral head is projected onto this area in normal anteroposterior (AP) radiographs. It is therefore difficult to diagnose femoral head necrosis from AP radiographs when changes are still minimal. Along with *axial* radiographs, we have had success in diagnosing such cases with *tangential* radiographs, as specified by Schneider (1970) (Fig. 1). A craniodorsal sector (30°) and two cranioventral sectors (30° and 60°) of the circumference of the femoral head are outlined using tangential radiographs. When they are used in conjunction with AP radiographs, a large section of the superior hemisphere of the femoral head can be surveyed. The necrotic area situated cranioventrally is shown most clearly in cranioventral tangential radiographs, which allow an earlier and more exact diagnosis than standard AP radiographs. In contrast, craniodorsal radiographs reveal a cranio-dorsal section of the femoral head, which is generally still in good condition. Tangential X-rays are therefore valuable not only for early *diagnosis* but also for a more accurate assessment of the *size* of the necrotic focus.

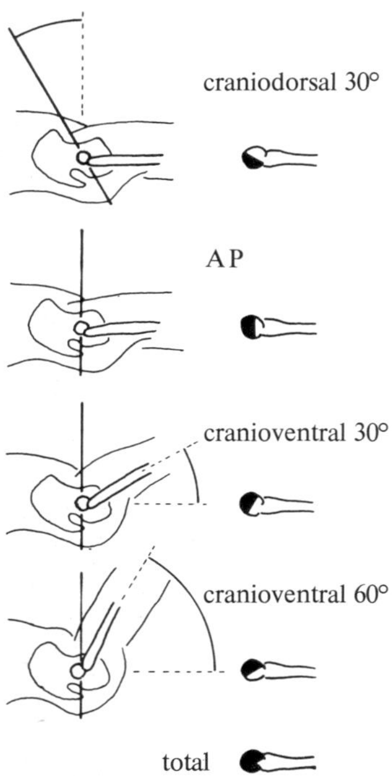

Fig. 1. Tangential views according to Schneider: four projection to demonstrate the femoral head radiologically. The craniodorsal sector is demonstrated by tilting the tube 30°; the cranial sector is shown on the AP view; and the cranioventral sectors are outlined by flexing the hip 30° and 60°. These four views permit interpretation of a relatively large area of the femoral head circumference

Principles of Treatment

As we have already confirmed (Willert and Sarfert 1975), *intertrochanteric femoral osteotomy with realignment of the femoral head* is definitely the procedure of choice among all presently available joint-preserving methods. This method may be assumed to have a favorable effect on the diseased joint in cases of segmental femoral head necrosis (similar to its therapeutic effect in coxarthrosis, Willert and Horrig 1979):

– Relaxation of the hip muscles (abductors, adductors, iliopsoas) and additional increase of the lever arm of the abductors reduce pressure on the joint and consequently on the necrotic segment (Pauwels 1960).

– Transposition of the femoral head transfers pressure onto a healthy section of the articular surface, thereby increasing the weight-bearing section of the circumference of the femoral head and relieving the necrotic segment from pressure and shear forces.

– Normalization of increased pressure in the medullary cavity. Immediate postoperative relief from pain, which is frequently observed, is attributed to this procedure (Arnoldi et al. 1971; Appel and Friberg 1973).

As the necrotic focus is located in the cranioventral segment of the femoral head, it can only be moved out of the acetabulum by anterior rotation. This is equivalent to extension of the femoral head. It is achieved when the distal fragment is flexed against the proximal fragment of the femur during osteotomy and the leg is extended at the hip after fixation of the osteotomy. As a rule, a healthy craniodorsal segment of the femoral head, instead of the loaded parts of the necrotic focus, is now located in the main weight-bearing area.

Flexion is usually combined with adduction of the distal femur during the osteotomy in order to cause varus alignment of the femoral neck-shaft angle. Fixation in internal rotation of the distal femur is advised to prevent a frequently observed alignment of the leg in an externally rotated position.

"Flexion osteotomy" has been used in cases of segmental femoral head necrosis since 1970, and highly favorable results have been repeatedly recorded since then (Willert and Sarfert 1974, 1975; Willert et al. 1977). The present study complements earlier reports by using a larger number of patients. Results have been critically evaluated once more.

Patient Material

Our paper is based on the follow-up results of 42 patients. In these cases, 51 hip flexion osteotomies were performed for segmental femoral head necrosis; nine patients therefore had bilateral operations (Table 1). Follow-up studies were carried out 5–81 months after the operation (Table 2). At the time of the operation, the patients' ages were 22–58 years, with an average of 39.5 years. Forty patients were men, two were women.

Changes or *conditions* associated with favoring the development of bone necrosis were as follows: Three patients had been treated with cortisone before hip changes had been noticed. One patient suffered from sickle-cell anemia, two from gout. Twelve patients were tentatively diagnosed as alcoholics, and in 32 patients lipid electrophoresis detected dyslipoproteinemia (Table 3). An increased transaminase level was found in 16 patients, and an increased fibrinogen level was present in 14 patients. None of our patients had had a previous trauma history.

Indications

No selection was used in performing flexion osteotomies. Flexion osteotomy was carried out on all patients with radiologically visible segmental femoral head necrosis, regardless of focal size, extent of collapse, or classification (Reichelt 1969). The only contraindication to flexion osteotomy was a hip flexion contracture of more than 10°. In these cases, we attempted to rectify the contracture by intensive preoperative physiotherapy.

Operative Technique

Radiological determination of the site of the necrotic focus showed with considerable consistency that flexion of approximately 30° allowed the most favorable adjustment of the femoral head. Additional varus correction of 10°–20° was performed, as well as internal rotation of 10°–20°.

Operations were carried out using instruments from the Swiss Association for the

Table 1. Compilation of hips with segmental femoral head necrosis arranged by clinical results (according to Fig. 4b)

#	Patient	Operated side	Age	Follow-up in months
1 (16)[a]	V.	left	46	32
2 (10)	H.	left	42	46
3	B. M.	right	46	49
4	C.	right	40	34
5	A.	right	38	32
6	K.	right	42	28
7 (9)	W.	right	49	30
8	Z.	right	39	33
9 (7)	W.	left	48	44
10 (2)	H.	right	43	38
11	W.	left	54	44
12	K.	left	44	81
13	L.	left	53	30
14 (15)	G.	left	34	51
15 (14)	G.	right	34	35
16 (1)	V.	right	50	14
17	S.	left	30	70
18	V.	left	36	20
19 (20)	W.	left	42	65
20 (19)	C.	right	51	19
21 (29)	M.	left	40	9
22	L.	left	58	18
23	K.	left	45	13
24	W.	right	31	24
25	A.	right	27	12
26	W.	left	38	19
27	C.	right	51	19
28	P.	right	30	60
29 (21)	M.	right	40	14
30	H.	left	41	28
31 (43)	B.	right	37	31
32 (33)	M.	left	32	27
33 (32)	M.	right	32	32
34	V.	right	39	24
35	P.	left	49	25
36 (46)	P.	right	30	16
37	G.	left	35	13
38	S.	right	40	21
39	W.	right	47	27
40	J.	right	52	32
41	K.	left	49	12
42	B. P.	right	29	26
43 (31)	B.	left	37	40
44	A.	right	54	13
45	K.	left	45	52
46 (36)	P.	left	31	7
47	P.	right	54	33
48	B.	right	38	60
49	S.	right	24	44
50	T.	left	26	22
51	S.	right	22	60

[a] The number in brackets refer to the contralateral side of patients with bilateral operations

Table 2. Period of follow-up observations in months after flexion osteotomy for segmental femoral head necrosis

Months	Number of hips	%
1–12	4	8
13–24	15	29
25–36	17	33
37–48	6	12
49–60	6	12
61–72	2	4
73–84	1	2

Table 3. Results of lipid electrophoresis in 32 patients

Dyslipoproteinanemia	Number
Fredrickson type II a	15
II b	2
IV	13
V	2

Study of Internal Fixation (AO). From a technical point of view, the operative procedure of flexion osteotomy resembles varus or valgus intertrochanteric osteotomy (Müller 1971, 1973) but the wedge is based anteriorly (Fig. 2). During varization, medial removal of some bone is also carried out simultaneously. The plate-seating instrument must be rotated by the size of the flexion angle against the longitudinal axis of the shaft (in our patients usually 30°) and be driven by the size of the varus angle in an ascending direction into the femoral neck. When the plate-seating instrument has been correctly positioned, it is possible to place the proximal osteotomy surface parallel to the instrument and the distal osteotomy surface at a right angle to the longitudinal axis of the femur. Care should be taken that the blade of the plate-seating instrument is not located too anteriorly.

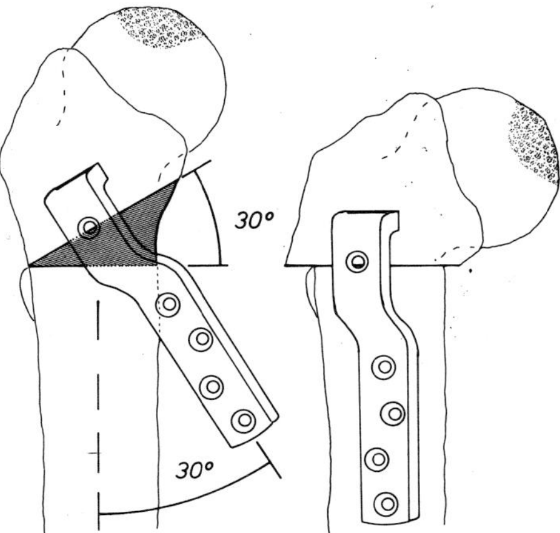

Fig. 2. Flexion osteotomy. The large cranioventrally located focus is rotated away from the weight-bearing area by removing a ventrally based intertrochanteric wedge of 30°. The osteotomy surfaces are then placed parallel to each other. (As a rule, valgization and internal rotation of the distal fragment is added to the flexion osteotomy. This is not shown in the drawing.)

Otherwise the anterior cortex of the femoral neck could be disrupted by the effect of leverage. It is essential to mark the rotation by drilling a Steinmann pin into the proximal and the distal fragment. If a flexion contracture persists despite preoperative physiotherapy, it is necessary to incise the anterior hip joint capsule and the iliofemoral ligament.

Postoperative Treatment

A short-leg plaster bed with a wooden bar is used postoperatively to avoid external rotation of the leg. After suture removal, hydrotherapy is instituted. Two to three weeks later, walking exercises are begun, and the operated-leg is protected from weight bearing by the use of forearm crutches. In cases of extensive areas of necrosis and even after consolidation of the osteotomy, we recommend that the patient continues to unweight the affected hip joint by using forearm crutches as long as possible. Careful physiotherapy is begun as active exercises 3 days postoperatively. After definite bony union of the osteotomy has occurred, intensive active and passive exercises are begun to improve the range of motion and remove contractures which may perhaps still exist. We did not use weight-reducing braces to relieve loading of the hip joint since their effect is doubtful (Wagner 1968).

Results

As in arthrosis therapy, the primary clinical aim in treating segmental femoral head necrosis consists of relieving the patient from persistent *pain* followed by improving *walking ability*. Improved joint motion is also desirable, although of less importance. From a morphological point of view, treatment aims at promoting revitalization of the necrosis, or at least at preventing progressive deformity of the femoral head. Great value is also placed on the patient's *subjective* comments, since it is ultimately he alone who can know and evaluate all the aspects which are important to *him*.

Clinical Parameters

Clinical parameters of pain, walking ability, and motion were assessed using the evaluation scale of Merle d'Aubigné et al. (1965), modified by Charnley (1968), with grade 1 (worst level) through grade 6 (optimal level).

Details of Individual Assessments (Fig. 3b)

Pain. The pain evaluation scale ranges from no pain at grade 6 to severe spontaneous pain at grade 1 (Table 4a). Starting with a preoperative pain assessment range from grade 1 to

Table 4a. Pain Grading

None	6	No pain or discomfort
Occasional	5	Occasional discomfort without limitation of activity
Slight	4	Discomfort during walking, but not during rest
Tolerable	3	Pain still tolerable, but activity is limited
Severe	2	Pain severe, marked limitation of activity
Very severe	1	Very severe, constant pain, even at night

Table 4b. Pre- and postoperative grading according to pain

Grading	Preoperative		Postoperative	
	Numbers	%	Numbers	%
"6"	–	–	15	29
"5"	1	2	21	41
"4"	10	19	7	14
"3"	30	59	5	10
"2"	9	18	3	6
"1"	1	2	–	–

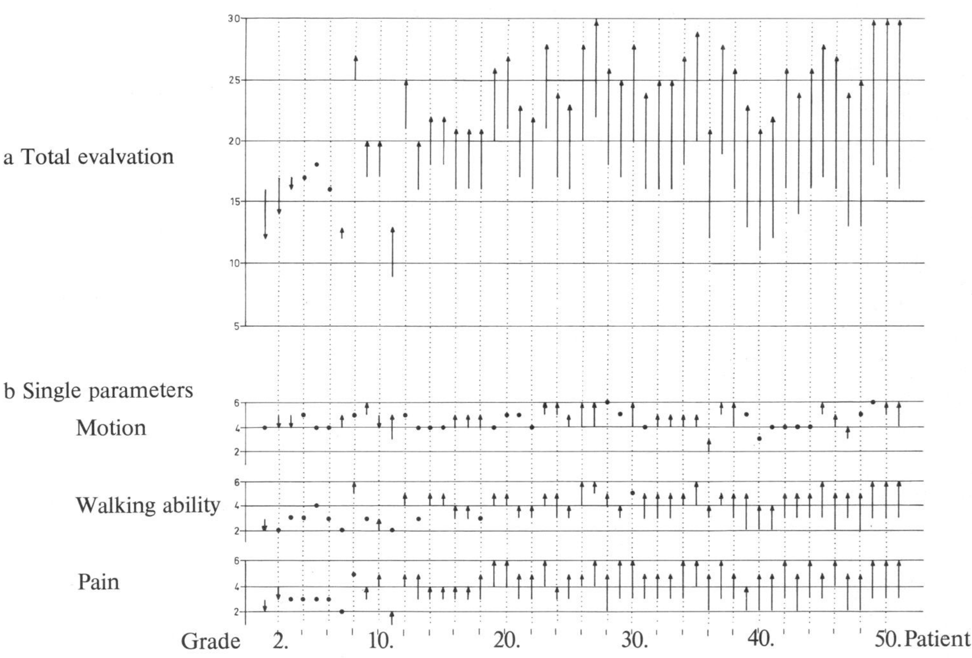

Fig. 3a, b. Representation of single parameters and total results of clinical evaluation data from follow-up examinations of 51 surgically treated hips, according to the classification of Merle d'Aubigné, modified by Charnley. Each hip is represented by an *arrow*, depicting preoperative values (base) and postoperative results (tip). A *point* means that no change occurred. **a** In the rubric *total evaluation*, findings for pain, walking ability, and motion are added together. According to their clinical importance, values for pain and walking ability were multiplied by two, values for motion by one. **b** In the rubric *single parameters*, values have been separated and shown without multiplication grade 5, 16 hips improved postoperatively by three grades, 17 hips by two grades, and 10 hips by one grade. This indicates improvement of 1–3 grades in 84% of operated hips.

Six hips remained unchanged, and two hips deteriorated further. At the time of the follow-up study, only eight hips were considered worse than grade 4 (mild pain) (Table 4b and Fig. 3b). In seven hips, persistent pain could be linked with radiologically visible focal enlargement and increasing "collapse" of the necrotic segment. Conversely, pain was no longer present in three hips, despite progressive radiological findings.

Walking Ability. The evaluation scale for walking ability ranges from normal, grade 6, to impossible, grade 1 (Table 5a). Postoperative evaluations of walking ability indicate improvement by three grades in 7 hips, by two grades in 13 hips, and by one grade in 19 hips. This signifies improvement of 1–3 grades in 76% of operated hips. The evaluation remained unchanged in 11 hips, and deterioration was found in only one hip. Patients frequently complained of initial discomfort after rest periods (Table 5b and Fig. 3b center).

Table 5a. Walking ability grading

Normal	6	Normal walking ability
Limp	5	Slight limp
One cane	4	Limp, patient requires cane for long distance walking
Reduced	3	Limited even with the aid of one cane, difficult without a cane
Limited	2	Walking time and distance with or without the aid of a cane is limited
Impossible	1	Patient is bed-ridden

Table 5b. Pre- and postoperative grading according to walking ability

Grading	Preoperative		Postoperative	
	Numbers	%	Numbers	%
"6"	–	–	8	16
"5"	3	6	22	43
"4"	12	23	10	19
"3"	27	53	7	14
"2"	9	18	4	8
"1"	–	–	–	–

Range of Motion. The range of hip joint motion was also evaluated on a scale of grade 6 (unrestricted) to grade 1 (almost totally restricted) (Table 6a). After realignment osteotomy, there was a two-grade improvement in the range of motion in only five hips, and a one-grade improvement in 18 hips. Twenty-five hips were unaffected, and deterioration occurred in three cases (Table 6b and Fig. 3b above).

Table 6a. Motion grading

211°–260°	"6"	Sum of	
161°–210°	"5"	Flexion – Extension	(max. 100°)
101°–160°	"4"	Abduction – Adduction	(max. 80°)
61°–100°	"3"	External rotation – Internal rotation	(max. 80°)
31°– 60°	"2"		260°
0°– 30°	"1"		

Table 6b. Pre- and postoperative grading according to motion

Grading	Preoperative		Postoperative	
	Numbers	%	Numbers	%
"6"	2	4	13	26
"5"	17	33	19	37
"4"	28	55	17	33
"3"	3	6	2	4
"2"	1	2	–	–
"1"	–	–	–	–

Overall Assessment

In order to form an overall picture of the effect of the disease on the health and functioning ability of the patients, the individual values of pain, walking ability, and range of motion can be documented to produce a relationship between preoperative and postoperative conditions (Figs. 3a, 4b). According to their clinical and functional importance, values for pain and walking ability were multiplied by two, while values for range of motion were multiplied by one. Therefore, the lowest possible value is grade 5 ($= 2 \times 1 + 2 \times 1 + 1 \times 1$), and the highest value is grade 30 ($= 2 \times 6 + 2 \times 6 + 1 \times 6$).

According to this assessment, improvement was found in 45 of 51 operated hips after flexion osteotomy, i.e., in 88%. There was no change in three hips (6%), and postoperative assessment showed deterioration in another three hips (6%). Of the improved hips 43, i.e., 84%, reached an overall evaluation of at least 20 which would correspond to an individual value of grade 4 in all the clinical parameters (mild pain, long-distance walking with one cane, overall range of motion 101°–160°). Twenty-six patients or 51% obtained an overall evaluation of at least 25, which corresponds to the second best grade 5 for each clinical parameter (Fig. 3a).

The range of improvement consists of 1–14 grades (Fig. 4b). In 36 hips (70%), there was at least one grade of improvement in each evaluation category; in 14 hips (27%), there was two-grade improvement. If the assessment of operative results is related to the range of clinical improvement, the following categories would be possible:

Unsatisfactory: improvement by 2 grades or less (8 hips)

Satisfactory: improvement by 3–6 grades (14 hips)

Good: improvement by 7–11 grades (25 hips)

Very Good: improvement by 12 grades or more (4 hips)

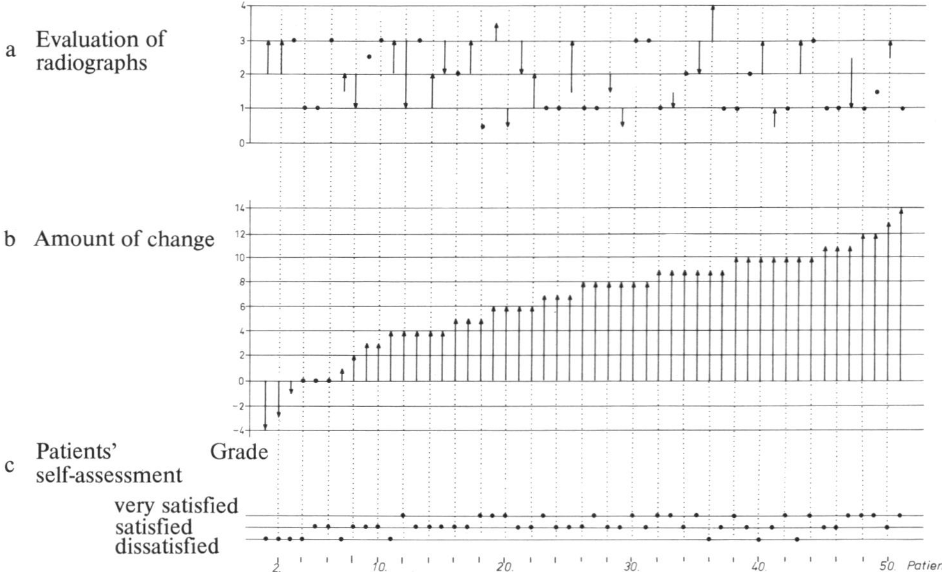

Fig. 4a–c. Juxtaposition of radiographic and clinical follow-up examination values and the patients' subjective postoperative assessment of 51 hips treated surgically, after Merle d'Aubigné, modified by Charnley. In **a** and **b** each hip is represented by an *arrow* depicting preoperative values (base) and postoperative results (tip). In **a** and **b** a *point* means that no change has occurred. In **c** the *point* represents the patients' subjective assessment. **a** Evaluation of the radiographs based on the size of the necrotic focus and the amount of collapse. **b** The *amount of change* is demonstrated by the length of the *arrow*, improvement or deterioration by its direction. Preoperative values were rated as 0 for better demonstration of the amount of change

Radiological Assessment

Radiological changes were assessed by determining the size of the necrotic segment and the extent of its collapse (Table 7). The least favorable assessment was used if different values for focal site and for collapse were present (Fig. 5).

Fig. 5a–c. Results of 51 hip flexion osteotomies in three-dimensions representation: **a** for pain, **b** for ▶ walking ability, **c** for motion, according to the classification of Merle d'Aubigné, modified by Charnley. Preoperative values are given on the *left*, postoperative values on the *right*. Each column represents a number of hips with similar assessment values. The results of our clinical follow-up examinations are coordinated with the preoperative values *within* the square. There each column represents the number of hips with similar pre- and postoperative assessment values. The front columns marked "Total" outside the square on the right side represent the number of hips with the same postoperative assessment values. The diagrams permit observation of postoperative results based on preoperative conditions. All hips on the left side of a diagonal transecting the square have deteriorated when compared to their preoperative condition. Hips touching the diagonal are unchanged. All hips on the right side of the diagonal have improved. Example: For the parameter "pain," 30 hips were rated preoperatively as 3. Postoperatively, one hip has deteriorated to grade 2, four hips were unchanged, six hips had improved to 4, ten hips to 5, and nine hips to 6

Pain
Total Preoperative assessment
Total Postoperative assessment
Walking ability
Range of motion
Deterioration
unchanged
Improvement
a
b
c

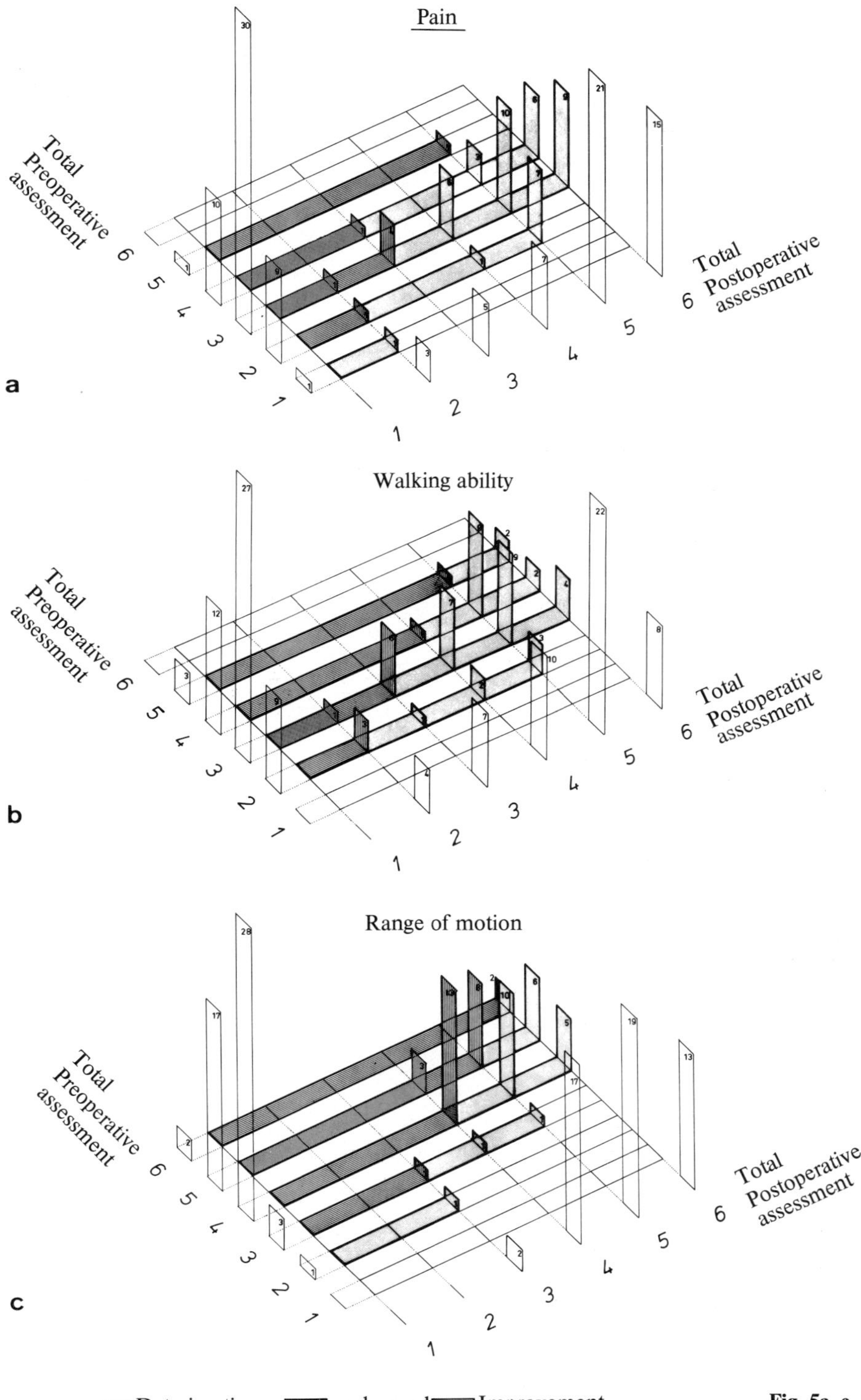

Fig. 5a–c

Table 7. Assessment criteria of radiologic serial observations

Focal size (in relation to the entire femoral head)	Grading	Collapse (in relation to the adjacent intact joint surface)
⅙	"1"	0 mm
¼	"2"	1 mm
⅓	"3"	2 mm
⅔	"4"	3 mm

Improved conditions were found in ten hips with partial focal consolidation. No change was noted in 24 hips; now and then increasing sclerosis was present in the necrotic area (Fig. 6). Focal size and depression increased in 14 hips (Fig. 7). During longer follow-up periods, arthrotic osteophytes appeared, which were all the more marked the larger the necrotic area. We could find no correlation between clinical improvement (Fig. 4b), the patients' subjective assessment of the results (Fig. 4c), and radiological observation of the course of the disease (Fig. 4a). For example, among patients with deteriorating radiological findings, two were very satisfied, five were satisfied, and only seven were dissatisfied (Fig. 8).

Occupational Rehabilitation of the Patient

The length of time our patients were unable to work clearly depended on their occupation. Patients involved in light manual labor resumed work much earlier than those involved in heavy manual labor. The length of time the patient was unable to work ranged between 1 and 12 months, with an average of 7 months. After the operation, 23 patients (55%) resumed the same occupation as before. Nine patients (21%) were retrained, and a further nine patients (21%) were still unable to return to work.

Fig. 6a–e. Radiological serial follow-up over a 5-year period after flexion osteotomy for segmental necrosis of the right femoral head (#28 in Table 1). Roentgenological evidence of slight enlargement and increasing structural changes of the necrotic focus of the right femoral head with cyst formation, sclerosis, and subchondral dissection, but without collapse of the necrotic segment. The joint space continues to be well-maintained. The *clinical* result is good, and the patient is subjectively satisfied. **a** preoperative: AP and axial view; **b** 1 year postop.: AP view; **c** 5 years postop.: AP view; **d** preop.: tangential views (Schneider); **e** 5 years postop.: tangential views (Schneider)

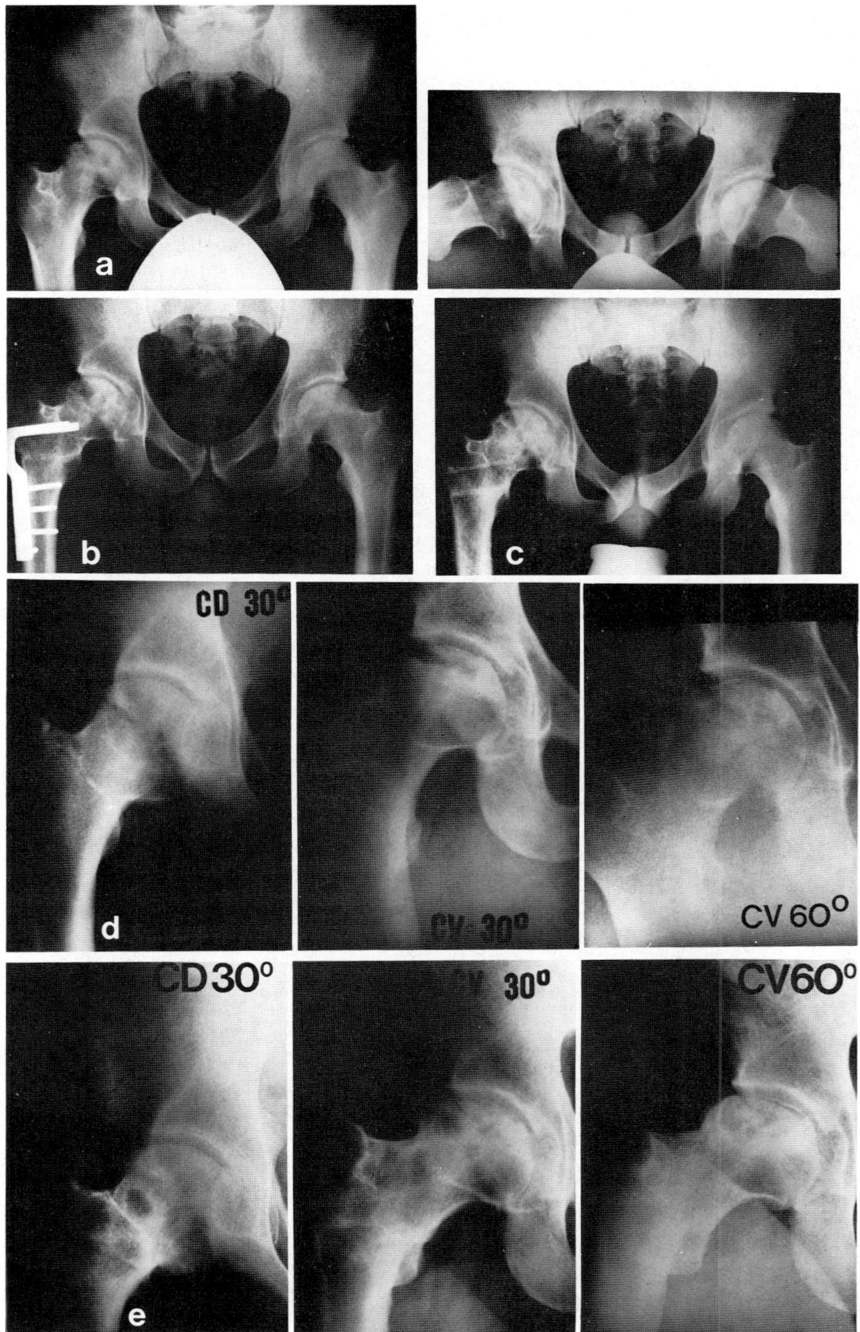

Fig. 6a–e

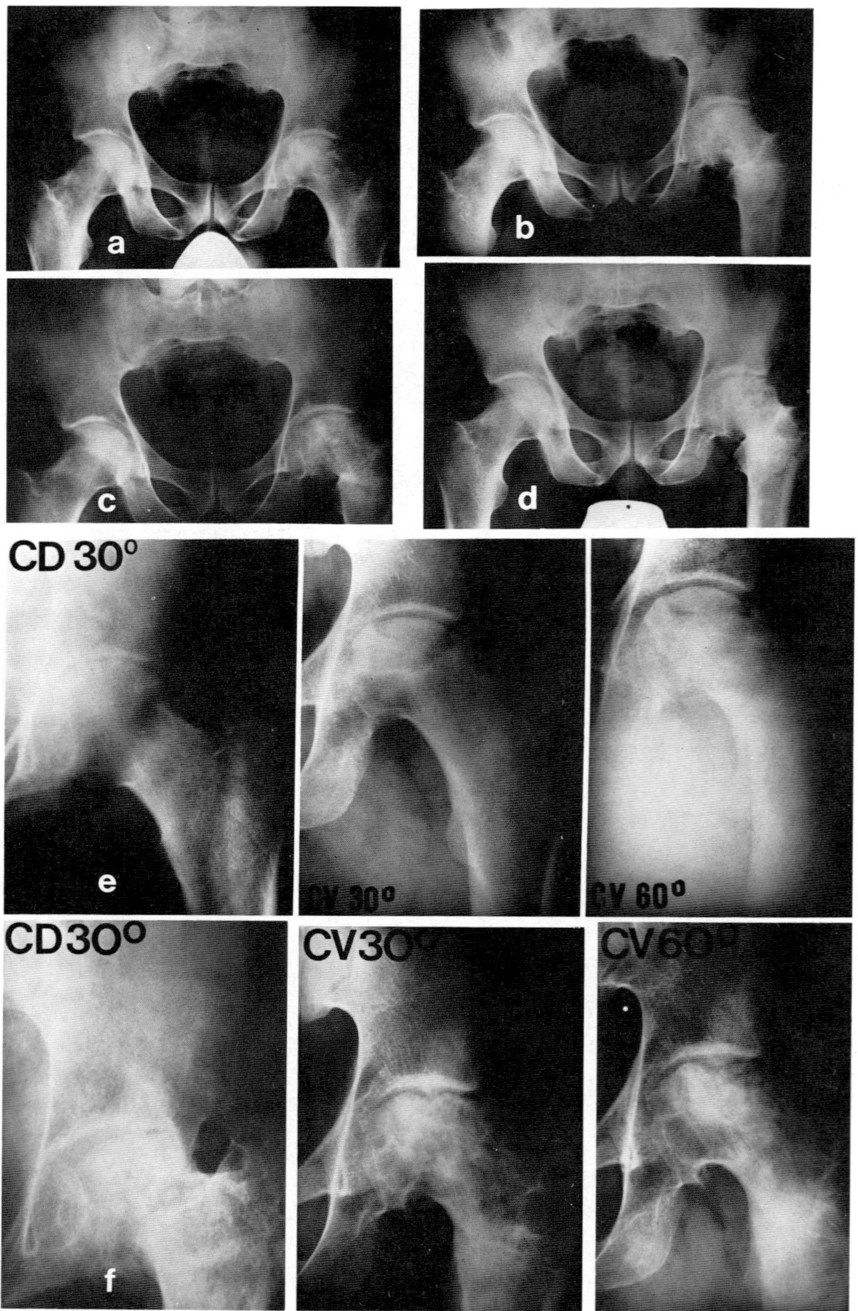

Fig. 7a–f

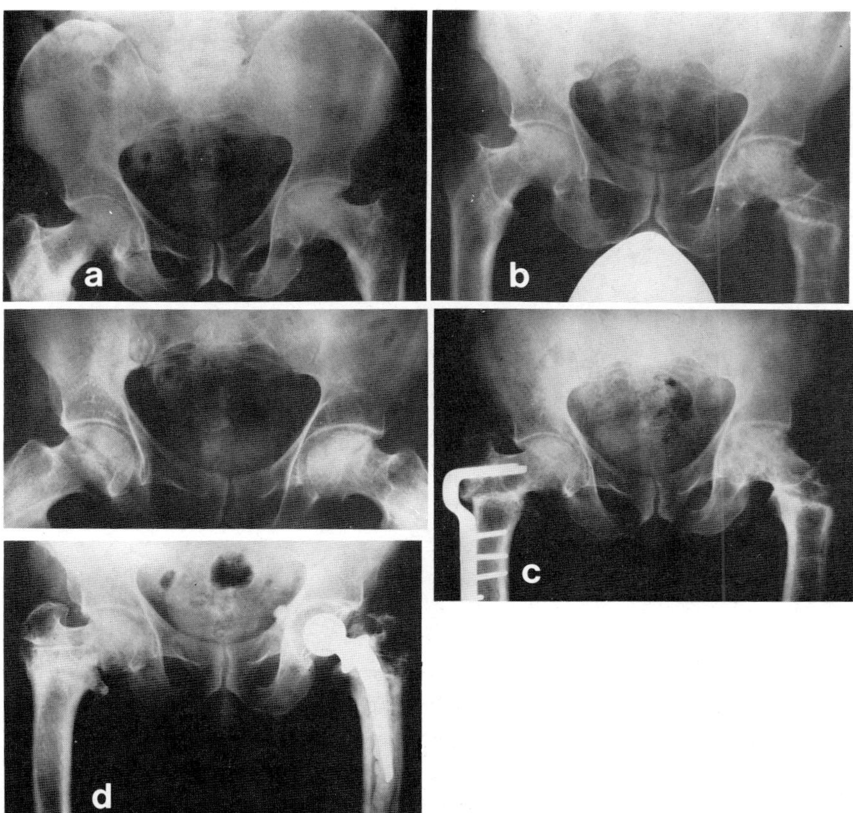

Fig. 8. Radiological serial follow-up after flexion osteotomy for bilateral femoral head necrosis. *Left*: (#1 in Table 1) After 4 years, marked roentgenologic evidence of structural changes in the necrotic focus of the femoral head without collapse of the necrotic segment. The joint space is maintained. The clinical result is poor; subjectively, the patient is dissatisfied. Total hip joint replacement with varus implantation of the femoral component. One year later, there is evidence of prosthesis loosening. The patient continues to have pain in his left hip. *Right*: (#16 in Table 1) Flexion osteotomy approximately 4 years after the operation on the left side. Follow-up examination 3 years later shows roentgenological evidence of increasing structural changes of the right femoral head without collapse of the necrotic segment. The joint space has become wider. The clinical result is relatively good; subjectively, the patient is more satisfied with his right hip than with the total joint replacement of the left hip. **a** Preop.: AP and axial view. **b** *Right*: 4 years after osteotomy of the left hip. Segmental necrosis of the right femoral head is now noticeable. *Left*: 4 years postop. **c** *Right*: 3 months postop. after flexion osteotomy. *Left*: 4 years postop. after flexion osteotomy. **d** *Right*: 3 years postop. after flexion osteotomy. *Left*: 1 year after left total hip joint replacement

---

◄ **Fig. 7a–f.** Radiological serial follow-up over a 7-year period after flexion osteotomy for segmental necrosis of the left femoral head (#17 in Table 1). Roentgenological evidence of slight enlargement and collapse of the necrotic focus with increasing degenerative changes and osteophyte formation at the craniolateral aspect of the femoral head. Fragmentation of the necrotic focus. Structural changes and sclerosis of the femoral head spongiosa. Slight diminution of the irregular joint space. The clinical result is still satisfactory, and the patient is subjectively satisfied. **a** preop.: AP view; **b** 3 years postop.: AP view; **c** 5 years postop.: AP view; **d** 7 years postop.: AP view; **e** preop.: tangential views (Schneider); **f** 7 years postop.: tangential views (Schneider)

Patients' Subjective Evaluation of Operative Results

Seventeen patients were "very satisfied" with the results of the operation, 25 were "satisfied," and 9 were "not satisfied." Eight of the dissatisfied patients were operated on 2.5–4.5 years ago, and an increase in the size of the necrotic area was shown by X-ray in five of these patients. Results considered unsatisfactory both from subjective and objective points of view were obtained particularly with older patients. Five of the unsatisfied patients were older than 45 years of age (Fig. 4c).

Complications

Direct complications of operative surgery included two cases of pseudarthrosis and one avulsion of the osteosynthesis plate. A total hip-joint endoprosthesis was implanted in two hips, once because of persistent pain and once because of pseudarthrosis.

Discussion

In general, quite good results were obtained from intertrochanteric "flexion osteotomy" in cases of segmental femoral head necrosis. Pain was relieved in 84% of cases, walking ability was improved in 76%, and range of motion was improved in 45%. Of the patients, 82% were satisfied or very satisfied with the results. Nevertheless, considerable discrepancies were evident between clinical evaluation, patients' assessments, and radiological evidence. In particular, clinical and functional results cannot be compared, or only very tenuously compared, with radiographs of the course of the disease.

It is remarkable that the favorable results were obtained on nonrandomized patients, since flexion osteotomy was performed on all cases with signs of segmental femoral head necrosis. Consequently, our experience shows that flexion osteotomy may be recommended as an operative treatment for segmental femoral head necrosis, since it provides a high percentage of satisfactory results and allows more or less pain-free use of the hip joint for as long as possible. Further measures, such as artificial hip joint replacement or arthrodesis, are still also quite possible (Fig. 8).

However, it must be emphasized that anatomical restoration of the changes cannot be obtained by realignment osteotomy at the proximal end of the femur. At best, this treatment may prevent further collapse of the necrotic area and progressive deformity of the femoral head. However, this did *not* occur in 27% of patients' hips which were treated. Consequently, there is no proof that relief from weight-bearing pressure favors revascularization of the necrotic segment. *In addition* to femoral head realignment, we therefore now prefer to remove as much as possible of the necrotic area and the fibrous demarcation zone through a window excised from the femoral neck. The resulting defect should be filled by a transplant of autologous spongiosa. Results obtained by this method so far are also good and very promising. However, it is still too early to compare this new combination therapy with flexion osteotomy, which has been practiced up to now.

Summary

This study reports on follow-up results of 51 flexion osteotomies performed in 42 patients for segmental femoral head necrosis. The follow-period ranged from 5 to 81 months. Pain was relieved in 84% of cases, walking ability was improved in 76%, and range of motion was improved in 45%. Subjectively, 82% of the patients gave positive evaluations of the results. However, in contrast, there are considerable discrepancies between objective and subjective clinical evidence on the one hand and the development of radiological findings on the other hand, since improvement of changes in the femoral head could be substantiated radiologically in only 20% of cases. However, since flexion osteotomy improves discomfort and function of the affected hip joint in a high percentage of cases and since it preserves an endogenous, mobile joint while still allowing subsequent measures to be taken, it can definitely be recommended as a form of therapy for segmental femoral head necrosis. For some time, simultaneous removal of the necrosis through the femoral neck has been practiced in addition to flexion osteotomy, and we hope that this will produce even better results in revascularization and regeneration of the necrotic area.

References

Appel H, Friberg S (1973) Effect of osteotomy on pain in idiopathic osteoarthritis of the hip. Acta Orthop Scand 44:710–718

Arnoldi CC, Lemperg RK, Linderholm H (1971) Immediate effect of osteotomy on the intramedullary pressure of the femoral head and neck in patients with degenerative osteoarthritis. Acta Orthop Scand 42:357–365

Charnley J (1968) The numerical grading of hips. Center for hip surgery, Wrightington Hospital, UK. Internal publication no 2

Fredrickson DS, Levy RI (1972) In: Stanbury JB, Wynngarden JB, Fredrickson DS (eds) The metabolic basic of inherited disease. 3rd edn McGraw-Hill, New York, chap 26

Merle d'Aubigné R, Postel M, Mazabraud A, Massias P, Gueguen J (1965) Idiopathic necrosis of the femoral head in adults. J Bone Joint Surg [Br] 41:612–633

Müller ME (1971) Die hüftnahen Femurosteotomien. Thieme, Stuttgart

Müller ME (1973) Intertrochanteric osteotomy in the treatment of arthritic hip joint. Surgery of the hip joint. Lea & Febiger, Philadelphia

Pauwels F (1960) Neue Richtlinien für die operative Behandlung der Koxarthrose. Verh Dtsch Orthop Ges 48

Reichelt A (1969) Die idiopathische Hüftkopfnekrose. Z Orthop 106:273–295

Schneider R (1970) Radiologische Funktionsdiagnostik zur Planung der intertrochanteren Osteotomie. Verh Schweiz Ges Orthop 131

Wagner H (1968) Ätiologie, Pathogenese, Klinik und Therapie der idiopathischen Hüftkopfnekrose. Verh Dtsch Orthop Ges 54:224–235

Willert HG (1977) Pathogenese und Klinik der spontanen Osteonekrosen. Z Orthop 115:444–462

Willert HG, Horrig C (1979) Alternativoperationen zum künstlichen Gelenkersatz bei Koxarthrose. Therapiewoche 29:8524–8537

Willert HG, Sarfert D (1974) Operative Behandlung der segmentalen Hüftkopfnekrose. Z Orthop 112:694–695

Willert HG, Sarfert D (1975) Die Behandlung segmentaler, ischämischer Hüftkopfnekrosen mit der intertrochanteren Flexionsosteotomie. Z Orthop 113:974–994

Willert HG, Zichner L, Enderle A (1977) Indikation und Ergebnisse der Flexionsosteotomie in der Behandlung der Hüftkopfnekrose. Z Orthop 115:484–485

Translation from the German: Willert H-G, Buchhorn G, Zichner L (1980) Ergebnisse der Flexionsosteotomie bei der segmentalen Hüftkopfnekrose des Erwachsenen. Orthopäde 9:278–289 © Springer-Verlag 1980

Treatment of Idiopathic Necrosis of the Femoral Head by Modified Cup Arthroplasty

Y. Gérard

It is our opinion that the treatment of idiopathic necrosis of the femoral head by femoral forage of the neck and evacuation of the necrotic bone is useful only at an early stage of the disease, before the onset of deformity of the head. Various methods of osteotomy have been described but, in our experience, these do not arrest the arthrosis which follows 4 or 5 years later. It appears illogical to perform a total hip arthroplasty if the acetabulum is healthy, and therefore it is our usual practice to perform an arthroplasty using a modified cup implant.

The cup is applied to the femoral head and gains purchase by resting against areas of healthy bone. Hemispherical cups tend to rotate into varus, and for this reason we prefer the pattern described by Luck (1970), which has a cylindrical form internally with respect to the femoral neck (Fig. 1). It is stable and can be utilized in all cases, except when the necrosis is massive (2% of our total series).

The operation is easy and can be performed through a small exposure, which does not compromise the blood supply to the femoral head. The femoral head must be reamed into a cylindrical shape of precise dimensions, and the axis must correspond strictly with that of the femoral neck. The alignment can be ensured by using the inferior border of the neck as a landmark, after excision of the inferior pole of the femoral head. The cup is driven onto the reamed femoral head, and nowhere does it touch the femoral neck.

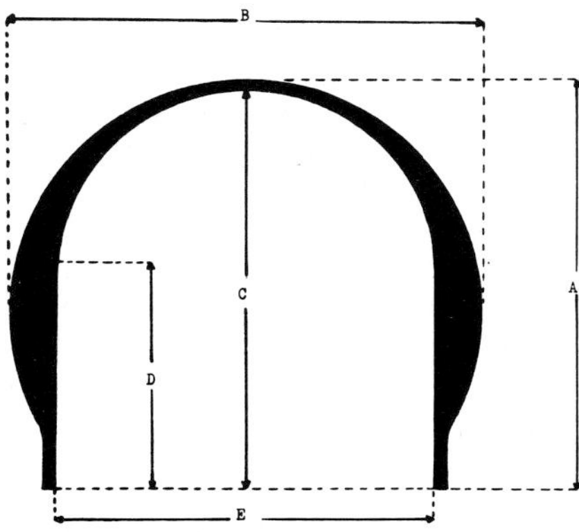

Fig. 1. Cup as modified by Luck, showing the cylindrical form for application to the femoral neck

Cement is not used. The dimensions of the cup are determined by the size of the acetabulum, and it is essential to have a complete range of sizes of cups at the time of operation. Postoperative progress is usually smooth; the patient is discharged after about 2 weeks and can resume work after about 3 months.

Since 1968 we have performed 105 Luck cup arthroplasties for idiopathic necrosis of the femoral head. We can report on 84 hips if we exclude those which have been operated on previously and those where the follow-up has not been sufficient. We shall record the results according to whether or not the idiopathic necrosis was accompanied by arthrosis at the time of operation.

Idiopathic Necrosis Without Arthrosis

There were 68 hips in which the idiopathic necrosis was not accompanied by obvious arthrosis at the time of operation. The follow-up period was at least 6 months.
Pain: Forty-four hips were pain free, 20 had occasional mild discomfort, perhaps associated with fatigue, and only 4 hips suffered more significant pain.
Range of motion: In 52 hips, flexion exceeded 90°, in 15 hips flexion was 70°–90°, and in 1 hip there was a contracture.
Gait: In 48 hips, gait was normal, while 18 experienced slight discomfort when fatigued, but were completely stable when weight-bearing was on the affected side. Only two cases were obliged to use a cane because of discomfort.

A general assessment using Merle d'Aubigné's method (1970) gave the following results:

Excellent: 31
Very good: 21
Good: 12
Fair: 1
Poor: 3
(Total: 68)

There were only four early failures; of these, three were associated with a technical error at surgery. In two of the latter, the cup was too large, and in the third, it was too small. These failures illustrate the importance of the availability of a complete set of cups at the time of operation. The fourth failure occurred in a very hyperlipidemic patient, who experienced pain which began during the first postoperative days and lasted until the time of follow-up. We do not know the reason for this continued pain.

The quality of the functional result obtained is important. A detailed study of 53 cases revealed that 37 had been able to return to their former work, three had had to change their work, three remained unemployed, two were retired but nevertheless able to pursue active lives, and eight remained disabled. Of the latter, two were disabled because of their hips and six because of other medical problems. These early good results have been maintained. It is of interest to speculate what changes occur in the stump of the femoral head and the reactions of the acetabular articular surface as a result of articulation with the cup.

Long-term observation has detected two clinical deteriorations in our cases. One of these occurred early, at about 10 months, and was due to a valgus disposition of the cup with respect to the neck. The other deteriorated in about the 2nd year and seemed to be associated with progression of the original condition of the femoral head. A study of the radiographs distinguishes possible deterioration with respect to the femoral or acetabular sides of the articulation.

On the femoral side, there were two definite instances in which the cup turned into varus; this led to a deterioration of the condition of the head beneath the cup. These two cases include the early deterioration in the hyperlipidemic patient mentioned above, while in the other patient there was clinical deterioration during the 2nd year.

In 13 cases there was a slight change in position of the cup. In 5, there was a sinking of the cup in line with the axis of the neck, and in 8, there were a few degrees of varization. These small displacements all occurred very early (in the first few months); after this, the

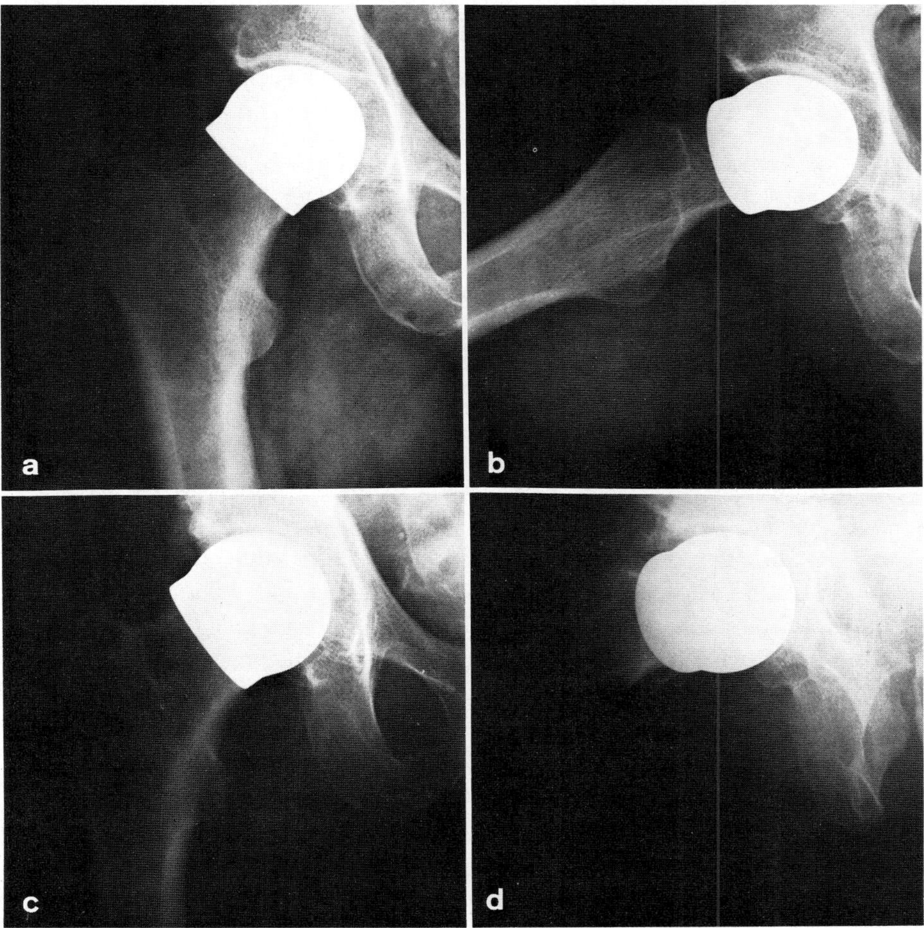

Fig. 2a–d. Patient B.A.G. (male, 45 years old). **a, b** anteroposterior and lateral radiographs immediately after operation; **c, d** anteroposterior and lateral radiographs 4 years after operation

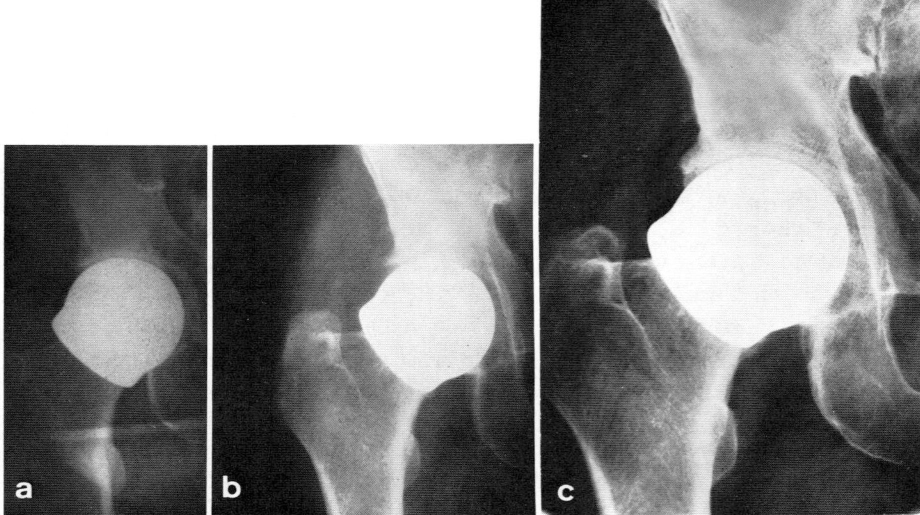

Fig. 3a–c. G.U.E. (male). **a** radiograph immediately after operation; **b** postoperative 6 months; **c** postoperative 7 years

cup position remained perfectly stable during the following years. There was no change in the clinical result, which remained satisfactory, and there was no associated deterioration in the condition of the femoral head. In certain instances, we have been able to detect bone growth in the region of the inferior edge of the femoral head over several years (Fig. 3), which helps to maintain the cup in position.

On the acetabular side, there were two other significant deteriorations. In one, there was a general narrowing of the joint space, which occurred towards the end of the 1st year and was associated with the cup in a valgus position and with lengthening of the neck of the femur. In the other, there was a narrowing which was related to the disease process itself; it equally affected the femur, and was observed in the 2nd year.

There were several minor deteriorations in the joint space; they occurred within 6–10 months after the operation, but there was no development of pain. This was seen in 3 of 42 cases, in which the acetabulum was thought to have been perfectly intact at the time of operation, and in 9 of 23 cases, where there had been a slight narrowing of the joint space before the operative intervention. It is of interest to note that even if there is a degree of wear of the articular cartilage, this can remain perfectly asymptomatic over several years of follow-up (Fig. 2). Contrary to the changes seen at the surface of a Moore-type prosthesis, there has never been any protrusion of the acetabulum with the modified cup arthroplasty. An adaptation of the acetabulum to the cup has been observed with development of osteophytes in the cotyloid fossa.

Idiopathic Necrosis Complicated by Arthrosis

This definition includes 16 cases, which occurred predominantly at the beginning of our series. The results are noticeably inferior to those in which there was no arthrosis at the time of operation. Without doubt, the results are completely satisfactory in three hips, with even the arthrotic changes disappearing during the months following insertion of the cup. However, in five hips there were poor results (31% of this group). We feel that the Luck cup arthroplasty, performed simply as described here, is not appropriate when an arthrosis is already present.

Conclusion

In 68 hips with idiopathic avascular necrosis, treatment was by a modified cup arthroplasty, in which the cup enclosed a cylindrically shaped femoral head. When no arthrosis had supervened by the time of operation, there were only six failures − four of these immediate and two delayed. Of the failures, three were certainly associated with technical errors at surgery and could have been avoided. Accordingly, the results in this group can be viewed favourably.

The early good results and their duration indicate that this procedure can be considered as one of the useful methods of management of necrosis of the femoral head. In our opinion, femoral forage should only be employed before X-ray changes are visible. Total prosthetic replacement or double-cup arthroplasty is necessary in cases where arthrosis has supervened. Similarly, in cases of massive destruction of the femoral head, a total prosthesis is necessary.

The most frequent type of case (stage 3 of Ficat) is that in which the sequestrated part has sunk or simply left a shell of unsupported cartilage over the surface. We believe that in such a case the modified cup has wide application and allows rapid recovery of activity of the hip; the result is maintained, lasting in this series for more than 8 years (Fig. 3).

References

Gérard Y (1973) Nécrose idiopathique de la tête fémorale. Traitement par cupule ajustée à appui cylindrique. Rev Chir Orthop [Suppl 1] 59:74–80
Gérard Y, Segal P, Bedoucha JS (1975) Traitement des nécroses idiopathiques de la tête fémorale par cupule ajustée à appui cylindrique. Rev Rhum Mal Osteoartic 42:275–285
Gérard Y, Segal P, Glavier B, Cuinet P (1979) La cupule ajustée à appui cylindrique. Traitement de choix de la nécrose idiopathique de la tête fémorale sans arthrose. J Chir (Paris) 116:487–492
Luck V (1970) Osteo-arthrosis of the hip characterized by progressive antero-laterale subluxation. J Bone Joint Surg [Am] 52:1271
Merle d'Aubigne R (1970) Cotation chiffrée de la fonction de la hanche. Rev Chir Orthop 56:481–486

Idiopathic Necrosis of the Femoral Head

Results of Intertrochanteric Osteotomy and Joint Resurfacing

H. Wagner and G. Zeiler

There are three reasons for the particular clinical importance of idiopathic femoral head necrosis:

1. When partial ischemic necrosis of the femoral head has spread to a greater or lesser extent, collapse of the articular surface results in severe damage to the hip joint.

2. Bilateral involvement often occurs, which considerably increases the extent of the disease yet simultaneously restricts the scope of treatment feasibilities.

3. The social significance of this disease is emphasized by the particularly frequent incidence of idiopathic necrosis of the femoral head in young men between the ages of 20 and 40. The disease results in severe, painful disability at the most active and most crucial time of life for professional advancement.

Idiopathic necrosis of the femoral head was previously a very rare, even virtually unknown syndrome, but over the past 20 years we have observed a steady increase of the disease described in publications and in our daily clinical practice. Besides the fact that better diagnostic methods may have resulted in an *apparent* increase of the syndrome, which in the meantime has become well-known and well-defined, we do not doubt that an *actual* increase in the syndrome may possibly be caused by changes in lifestyle. For example, there has been a marked increase of alcoholics among our own patients over the past 10 years.

Etiology, Pathogenesis, and Clinicoradiological Development

Even today, still relatively little is known about the etiology of so-called idiopathic necrosis of the femoral head. Published opinion concurs that necrosis is produced by occlusions in the terminal vascular system of the craniolateral segment of the femoral head and that there is a striking concomitant incidence of arthritis urica, liver parenchyma damage, or chronic alcohol abuse. Sickle-cell anemia is frequently found in black patients with femoral head necrosis. Necroses of the femoral head are also observed in cases of chronic polyarthritis, caisson disease, long-term administration of corticoid preparations and Cushing syndrome, which are indistinguishable from idiopathic necrosis. In the past 10 years, reports of idiopathic necrosis of the femoral head have also been published in conjunction with lipometabolic disorders (Boettcher et al. 1970; Eichler 1974;

Liebig and Weseloh 1977, Merle d'Aubigne et al. 1965; Patterson et al. 1964; Pohl 1971; Zsernaviczky et al. 1976), and increase of intramedullary pressure has been described (Ficat and Arlet 1977; Hungerford, personal communication 1975, 1979).

Compared with this, there are no known figures to ascertain the frequency of femoral head necrosis in the syndromes mentioned (arthritis urica, alcoholism, etc.). However, since idiopathic femoral head necrosis actually occurs more frequently in these disorders, their pathogenetic significance cannot be casually dismissed.

There are manifold courses of idiopathic necrosis of the femoral head. Many patients complain of very severe initial pain, which may radiate from the groin along the inner side of the thigh to the knee joint. Radiographs taken at that time show no evidence of disease. Pain eases after a few days, but slowly recurs after 8–12 weeks with increasing intensity, in correlation with the amount of weight-bearing pressure. Radiographs may now show the first important early sign of a necrotic area on the ideal spherical shape of the femoral head. This is a thin, wavy radiolucent line corresponding to the subchondral defect created by separation of the still intact articular cartilage from the underlying necrotic bone (Fig. 1). Often only lateral radiographs reveal this phenomenon.

Despite periodic variations and an initial good response to symptomatic medications and physiotherapy, hip discomfort slowly increases as the disease progresses, depending on the amount of weight-bearing pressure. After a few more weeks radiographs reveal the second important early sign, when the femoral head begins to lose its spherical shape. Long before a demarcation appears between the necrotic segment of the femoral head and the surrounding bone structure, a very slight collapse of the articular surface takes place over the necrotic area, which can be detected by Müller's ischiometer (Fig. 2).

As the disease progresses, there is more discomfort due to weight-bearing pressure and increasing limitation on abduction and internal rotation of the hip joint. Due to collapse of the necrotic area, a ridge appears on its anterior margin in the articular surface, which may result in painful pinching of the limbus. Radiographs now show an increasing

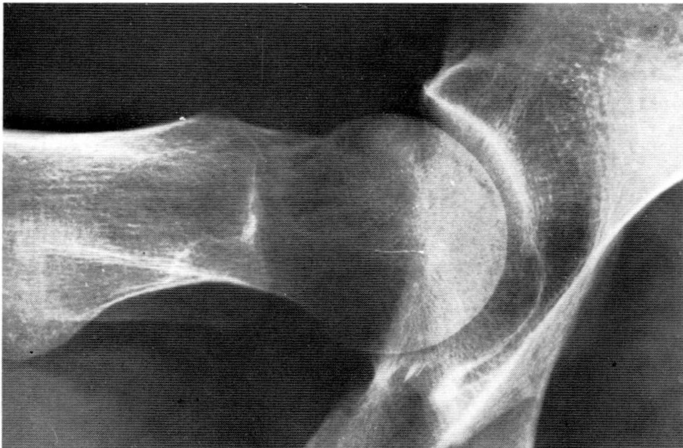

Fig. 1. Subchondral radiolucent line on the femoral head in idiopathic femoral head necrosis (lateral radiograph). The radiolucent line corresponds to the buffer zone between the immediate subchondral layer of bone and the necrotic segment of the femoral head

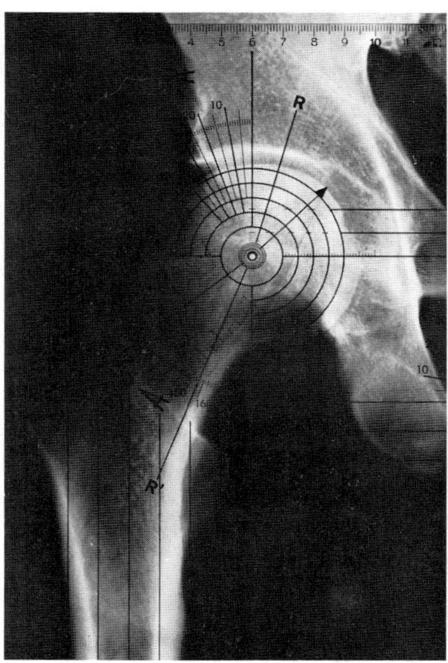

Fig. 2. Müller's ischiometer shows slight flattening of the cranial segment of the femoral head in idiopathic femoral head necrosis

line of demarcation between the necrotic area and the surrounding bone. At the interface with the necrosis, living osseous tissue becomes compacted, whereas on the corresponding surface of the necrotic area, resorption processes take place until the entire circumference of the necrotic area is detached from its original contact with its bony surroundings. Consequently, the focus also loses its stability. This results in progressive collapse of the bony necrotic focus and the overlying articular surface and in its painful relative movement against the surrounding bone caused by weight-bearing and movement. On the focal margin, folds and cracks are formed in the articular cartilage (Fig. 3). Due to progressive resorption of the necrotic bone, the slight depression of the articular surface becomes increasingly deeper, until finally the acetabular rim penetrates the articular surface defect. This consequently results in lateralization of the femoral head (Fig. 4) with adduction contracture of the hip joint and functional shortening of the leg.

In many patients, femoral head necrosis develops imperceptionally without the attacks of pain described above. Patients first become aware of their illness because of slowly increasing discomfort caused by weight-bearing forces and by decreased joint motion. Radiographs taken at this point usually reveal an advanced stage of femoral head necrosis. Occasionally patients are observed who have experienced no pain at all for a long period of time. In these cases a radiological examination, performed for slight temporary discomfort, may reveal extensive, subtotal, bilateral necrosis of the femoral head (Fig. 5).

Hip pain depends on the width of the radiological joint space, the mechanical stability of the necrotic area, and the nature of impediments to interarticular movement. A thick layer of articular cartilage with interspersed compact scar tissue can act as an effective buffer for uneven articular surfaces over a long period of time if the joint space is wide. More severe discomfort can thus be prevented for years. In a narrow joint space, where

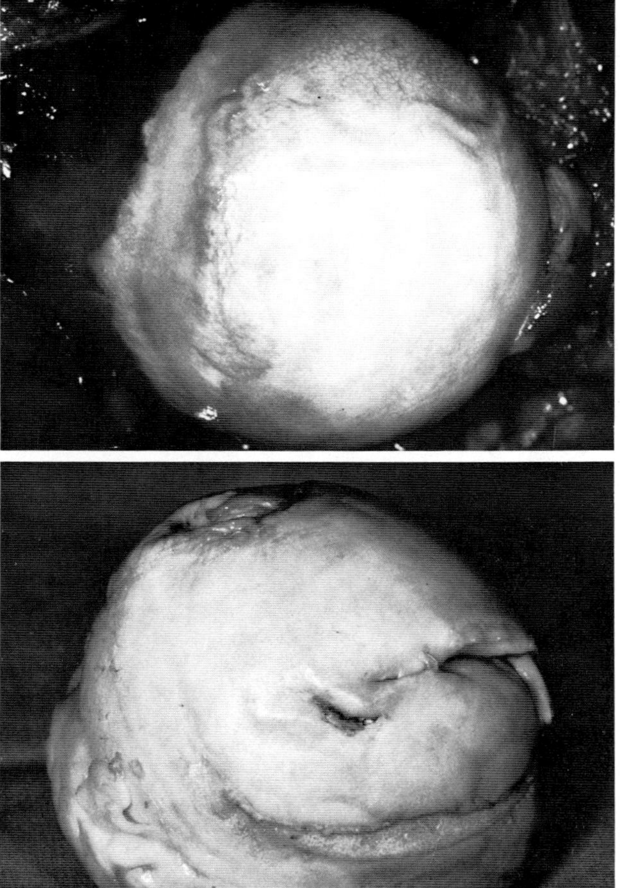

Fig. 3. Different stages of articular surface deformity in idiopathic necrosis of the femoral head. *Above*: Slight collapse of the articular surface segment with ridges forming in the articular cartilage. *Below*: Advanced stage with flap-like cracks in the articular cartilage and marked arthrotic reaction

the buffer layer is already worn down, unevenness of the articular surface and sharp-edged defect ridges cause severe friction phenomena which perpetuate painful irritation. Painful mechanical irritation is also caused by a necrotic area that is unstable because it is undermined by a wide resorption zone or is cracked or softened. Weight-bearing with very little discomfort may be guaranteed for a long period if the necrotic focus has collapsed as a coherent solid block or if it is tightly wedged into the substratum, thus ensuring stability. Ridges on the articular surface at the focal margins do not necessarily result in pain. This depends on their localization and on other mechanical details. This fact is the basis for the effectiveness of an intertrochanteric osteotomy. With this operation we do not remove an articular surface irregularity, but we position it in a different area and thereby obtain immediate alleviation of pain.

In all different types and degrees of severity of idiopathic necrosis of the femoral head, the lateral margin of the femoral head that continues into the lateral cortex of the femoral

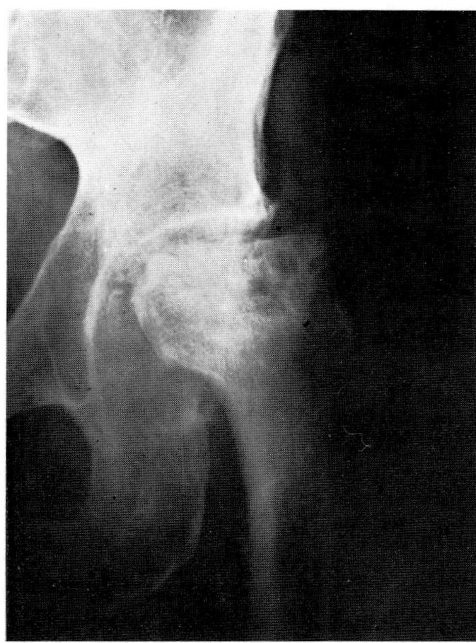

Fig. 4. Advanced idiopathic necrosis of the femoral head with extensive collapse of the articular surface, collapse of the acetabular roof into the femoral head defect, and marked lateralization of the femoral head

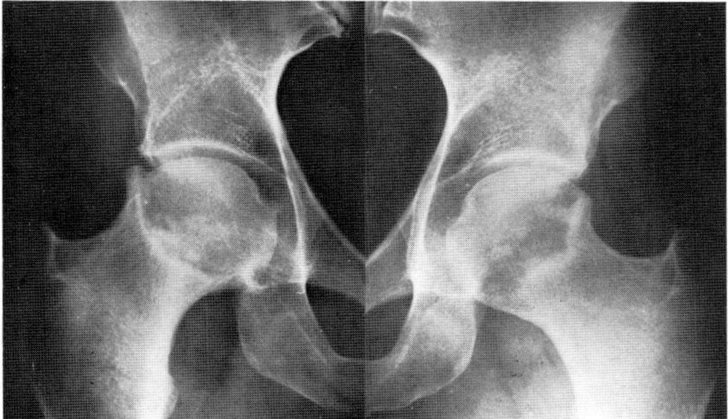

Fig. 5. Extremely severe bilateral subtotal necrosis of the femoral head in a 36-year-old woman. Despite massive necrotic changes and almost total collapse of the articular surface of the right femoral head, the patient has no appreciable discomfort since mechanical stability is still present

neck is always preserved and consists of particularly solid, hyperemic bone of good quality. This is important for the anchoring of a resurfacing prosthesis.

The size of necrotic areas frequently concurs with other clinical findings, a fact rarely mentioned in the literature, even though it can be extremely helpful in our attempts at diagnosis. Only a few of the findings shall be mentioned here. For example, in patients with very extensive necrosis of the femoral head, we find striking premature aging, a tendency to be overweight, and marked capillary ectasias on the cheeks above the zygomatic arches and also occasionally on the sides of the nose; vascular fragility with hematoma formation even after slight contusions is frequent. In these relatively young people, skin elasticity is lost, and the subcutaneous fatty tissue has a puffy appearance. Alcoholics with extensive necrosis of the femoral head usually have a pale complexion and a pre-cachetic reduction in their general state of health. Intraoperatively, we observed in both groups that there were decreased water-binding properties of collagenous tissue with rapid dehydration of skin and fasciae at the wound surface. The fascia lata has very often a slightly yellow color, which is not found in other hip diseases.

The basic causes of these clinical observations, which we could continue to enumerate at length, are still largely unknown. However, they are a further indication that in cases of idiopathic femoral head necrosis we are not dealing with a localized lesion but with a systemic disease which only affects the precarious part of the skeleton, the "femoral head", in this particular way.

The various types of progression of idiopathic femoral head necrosis described illustrate how difficult it can be to arrive at an early diagnosis of this syndrome, the more so since the majority of patients do not seek medical advice until advanced changes have occurred. Conversely, in all publications there is unanimous demand for early diagnosis since this enables one to obtain better results.

From a practical medical point of view, one must question whether such a request can be upheld since it cannot be fulfilled in the majority of cases, due to the late onset of discomfort and the belated action by the physician. In this connection one also has to ask if very early diagnosis of idiopathic femoral head necrosis would actually influence the results of treatment and at which stage of the disease it is best to begin operative treatment.

Basic Ideas on Therapy

Hungerford (personal communication 1975, 1979) argues that imminent femoral head necrosis can be recognized by the increase in intramedullary venous pressure. He postulates that irreversible bone infarction can be prevented if pressure is released by previous drilling of the medullary canal. If this is true, the earliest diagnosis possible is extremely important, but it will be difficult to quantify the therapeutic effect if necrosis has not yet occurred.

In the large number of patients in whom manifest avascular necrosis is already present at the first examination, other aspects are important. The earliest possible diagnosis is also desirable in these cases, but the question arises as to whether a delayed diagnosis is necessarily disadvantageous for the patient. There is no definite evidence that early treatment will limit the necrotic focus to a smaller area and that delayed treatment allows the necrosis to spread to a larger area. On the contrary, all observations point to the fact that the size of the necrotic focus is determined from the beginning and that the actual extent of the necrosis is fully revealed only during the gradual process of demarcation.

This has practical clinical consequences: When an osteotomy to preserve the joint is to be considered, the operation should not be delayed until severe changes in configuration and arthrotic reactions have occurred in the hip joint. The operation should rather be proposed before secondary changes have developed, since a better condition of the articular surface permits a more favorable prognosis for the osteotomy. On the other hand, when femoral head necrosis has been diagnosed very early, an osteotomy should not be performed immediately but should be delayed until the *initial* process of demarcation permits a reliable assessment of focal size. Demarcation is still the most important criterion today, since indications for intertrochanteric osteotomy actually depend on the extent of necrosis and since reliable assessment of focal size is not possible by bone scans and tomographic examination during the early stages. Performing an osteotomy too early, based on an under-assessment of the extent of the focus, will necessarily end in failure.

When very large necrotic areas are present and only joint replacement or occasionally an arthrodesis is indicated, an early operation should also not be considered. It should be delayed until pain, malposition and functional loss, or increasing bone atrophy make operative intervention unavoidable.

Choosing the correct time for surgery is indeed very difficult and requires much experience. If a decision is made to postpone the operation on the basis of clinical findings and negligible discomfort, careful clinical and radiologic follow-up examinations are required so that, despite the slight amount of discomfort, morphological changes which could limit future possible methods of treatment do not by chance occur. In general one should consider indications for different treatment modalities very critically, weighing the expected outcome against the magnitude of the contemplated operation. Negligible improvement of the situation at the expense of a major operation is a disproportionate solution. In particular, when performing joint-preserving osteotomies, one has to analyze possible future developments, so that a failed osteotomy does not worsen the prospects for joint replacement. On the other hand, the effectiveness of an osteotomy must be given its proper value, so that a relatively young patient does not undergo joint replacement when he could have benefited from an osteotomy for 10 or 15 years. In order to gain time for patients who experience little discomfort, one should consider early surgical intervention and, above all, a joint replacement, only if surgery at a later date would lead to a less successful result.

Hip Arthrodesis

Despite the fact that many patients are young, arthrodesis of the hip joint is only considered very rarely in the treatment of femoral head necrosis for the following reasons. We know from experience that the rate of bony union of an arthrodesis, even when one uses modern methods of stable osteosynthesis, is delayed in cases of idiopathic femoral head necrosis. Reoperations are required more frequently than in other hip disorders due to implant breakages, secondary malalignment, or complaints due to instability. In addition, recovery is prolonged, which considerably reduces the appeal of this method of treatment.

However, a far more important restraint against this method is the fact that idiopathic femoral head necrosis often occurs bilaterally, which prohibits the use of an arthrodesis as a primary procedure. When bilateral hip damage occurs, at least one hip joint must be preserved. The prospect of saving function is doubled if initially both joints are kept movable. It has to be accepted that all presently available measures to preserve or replace a joint in the presence of severe changes are only a temporary and limited solution. When bilateral involvement occurs, arthrodesis should be the last resort after previous operations have failed to preserve function.

In cases of bilateral hip joint involvement, the old rule of creating a stance leg by arthrodesis and then trying one's best to preserve motion in the other hip joint has severely restricted the range of therapy and has therefore not been successful. Preserving motion in both hip joints initially has proved its worth, even when considering the problems and temporary limited effectiveness of hip operations which are presently available to preserve motion. Arthrodesis can still be considered at a later date if steps to preserve motion failed in one of the hip joints. A primary arthrodesis might, after all, cause fusion of that hip joint in which preservation of function would actually have been more successful.

The fact that arthrodesis is very poorly accepted by patients should not be disregarded. Good hinge motion usually still exists, even in cases of idiopathic femoral head necrosis where advanced changes in the shape of the femoral head and severe weight-bearing discomfort are present. As soon as preoperative pain is forgotten, patients perceive arthrodesis as an unpleasant loss of function, which is not outweighed subjectively by painfree weight-bearing.

The important role of technology in our lives also contributes in part to further reasons for the negative attitude towards hip arthrodesis. For example, patients can avoid extensive walking, which was previously considered so important, by using modern transportation. Moreover, hip arthrodesis renders the use of cars, trains, or airplanes far more difficult. After hip arthrodesis, it is difficult for a person taller than 175 cm to use a car.

On the whole, performing a hip arthrodesis should be considered with greater reticence today than in former times, since better alternative methods are now available and the negative effects of fusing the hip joint are better known. Even today there is no doubt that arthrodesis provides a lifelong, load-stable, and practically risk-free solution for the painful, diseased hip joint. However, relief is only provided for the fused hip joint, whereas abnormal loading causes new problems for the vertebral column, the knee joint on the same side, and the contralateral hip joint. These problems become evident 15–20 years later.

However, the most important reservation against primary hip joint arthrodesis is the fact that joint-preserving osteotomies and alloplastic joint replacements are so efficient today that arthrodesis should no longer be seriously considered. Therefore, in our therapy arthrodesis of the hip joint should be considered as the last rather than the first step.

Subchondral Spongiosa Plasty

Subchrondral spongiosa plasty was previously performed by us quite frequently when experience in treating idiopathic femoral head necrosis was still very limited (Wagner 1967). In this procedure, the hip joint is exposed through an anterior or anterolateral approach and, after subluxation of the femoral head, the subchondral focus is removed.

The resulting defect is filled with autologous spongiosa from the iliac crest. If the articular cartilage is still intact at the time of surgery, the focus is undermined and filled through the border of the femoral head. If, on the other hand, cracks are already present in the articular cartilage on top of the focal margin, the articular cartilage is lifted up in a flap-like fashion, and the focus is removed through the articular surface. The main advantage of this procedure is that the collapsed cartilaginous articular surface can be elevated.

As the necrotic areas of the femoral head are surrounded by very compact, living, hyperemic bone, it is not surprising that spongiosa grafts are well incorporated into such foci. Immediate pain relief is also impressive. It is due both to the mechanical solidification of the articular surface at the focal area by the supporting spongiosa graft and to the smoothing of the articular surface ridges on top of the focal margin. After 3 months of functional treatment involving careful partial weight-bearing, good loading capacity is obtained in small to medium-sized foci.

However, since the foci are located in a heavily loaded area of the joint, further gradual collapse of the articular surface near the focus is inevitable, even after careful elevation of the articular surface and thick padding with spongiosa. Consequently, incongruence persists in the main weight-bearing area of the hip joint. Nevertheless, it is impressive that after spongiosa grafts have been incorporated, patients may live for many years with very little discomfort and good function (Fig. 6).

Good results were obtained using subchondral spongiosa plasty on foci measuring up to 25 mm in diameter in patients who were followed more than 15 years after the operation. Subchondral spongiosa plasty is overtaxed by foci measuring more than 25 mm. In this case, secondary deformities soon recur with unsatisfactory clinicoradiologic results, due to the large extent of revascularization and the relatively large section of the articular surface occupied by the focus.

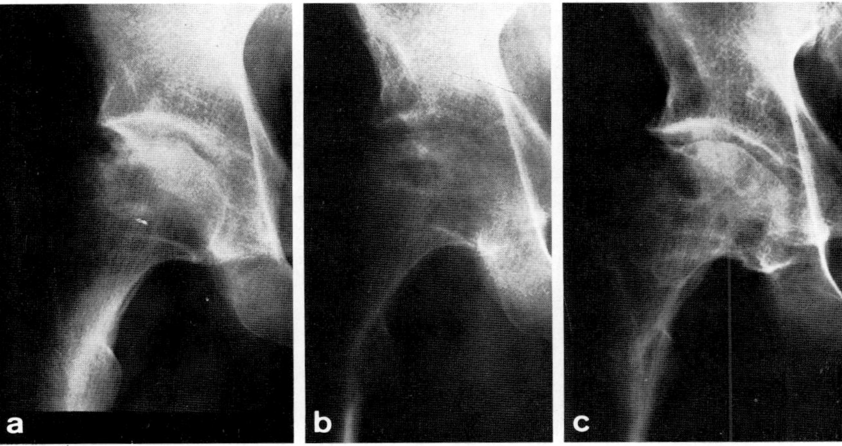

Fig. 6a–c. Subchondral spongiosa plasty for idiopathic necrosis of the femoral head in a 35-year-old man. **a** Preoperative radiograph. **b** Six weeks after subchondral spongiosa plasty with marked reactive bone atrophy in the area of the hip joint caused by the operation and relief from weight-bearing. **c** Sixteen years after subchondral spongiosa plasty. Despite deformity of the articular surface, a wide joint space exists with good hinge motion and slight discomfort during long walks

One important disadvantage of subchondral spongiosa plasty is that the operative technique and postoperative physiotherapy are relatively difficult and complicated procedures. An eye-opening observation was made in our own clinic in that subchondral spongiosa plasty has been gradually replaced over the years by intertrochanteric osteotomy for patients with comparable initial findings and that good results were also obtained by younger surgeons using this simpler method.

In conclusion, therefore, subchondral spongiosa plasty performed on necrotic foci measuring up to 25 mm in diameter causes the femoral head defect to be filled with osseous tissue. However, equally good results can be obtained more easily by intertrochanteric, flexion-valgus osteotomy.

Ganz and Noesberger (1978) recently introduced a combination of subchondral spongiosa plasty with intertrochanteric osteotomy. We have performed this procedure so far only in specific cases as a two-stage operation. Ganz substantiates the reason for this extension of surgical intervention by stating that, despite functional improvement due to intertrochanteric osteotomy alone, reossification of the necrotic focus of the femoral head proceeds very slowly or is actually absent, whereas an additional spongiosa plasty results in a quicker filling of the femoral head defect with bone.

Homologous Articular Surface Transplantation

Homologous articular surface transplantation had been previously performed by us in special cases in young patients with severe articular surface defects (Wagner 1972). However, there is no longer any indication to perform this extensive operative procedure for idiopathic femoral head necrosis since good results have been obtained in the meantime with intertrochanteric osteotomy on the one hand and resurfacing on the other hand. Moreover, we have realized that articular surface transplantation of the femoral head and acetabulum offers only a temporary and limited solution. Equally good results may be obtained with less effort by osteotomy or resurfacing.

Presently the indication for transplanting an articular surface and the femoral head is given in cases of posttraumatic partial femoral head necrosis with articular surface collapse in young patients where the articular surface of the acetabulum is well-preserved, provided that lateralization of the femoral head does not require the need for pelvic osteotomy (Wagner 1978b).

Intertrochanteric Osteotomy

Intertrochanteric osteotomy, which we generally practice in the form of flexion-valgus-rotation osteotomy, is, in our experience, the most universal and numerically the most significant method of treatment. The functional mechanisms of intertrochanteric osteotomy have always been described in the following way. The involved area of the articular surface of the femoral head is transferred away from the main loading region by rotation

of the femoral neck and head. Consequently, a healthy area of the femoral head is transferred by rotation into the main weight-bearing zone. This correction is in fact far more
complex and causes simultaneous changes in several components of the hip joint.

First of all, it should be stated that, due do its extent, the necrotic focus cannot usually
be completely rotated out of the weight-bearing area by intertrochanteric osteotomy. To
accomplish this, a greater angle of correction is required than is possible with intertrochanteric osteotomy. In 1967 Wagner presented a double intertrochanteric osteotomy
for more extensive correction (Fig. 7, 8) in which the femoral neck is rotated on its
longitudinal axis until the necrotic area completely disappears from the hip joint, and
only truly healthy sections of the articular surface of the femoral head are in contact with
the cranial articular surface of the acetabulum. Several years later, Sugioka (1973) described an anterior transtrochanteric rotation osteotomy of the femoral neck to reach the
same goal. In contrast to double intertrochanteric osteotomy, the transtrochanteric
osteotomy, which is performed at the base of the femoral neck, has the disadvantage that
it endangers the arterial blood supply of the femoral neck and head due to anatomic conditions at the fossa trochanterica. Moreover, reliable, exercise-stable osteosynthesis is
doubtful because of the short femoral neck fragment. At any rate, better correction does
not follow.

However, clinical experience has shown that such extensive corrections, which can be
accomplished by intertrochanteric double osteotomy or transtrochanteric rotation
osteotomy, are by no means required for idiopathic necrosis focus. Our goal is to rotate
the necrotic focus away from the *center* of the weight-bearing area and to locate a healthy,
spherical section of the articular surface of the femoral head in the vertex of the joint. For
this reason, apart from cases of severely deformed congenital dislocations of the hip joint,
we have no longer performed double intertrochanteric osteotomies for idiopathic
femoral head necrosis in recent years (Wagner 1977).

Since the necrotic focus is necessarily located in the anterosuperior segment of the
femoral head, it lies in the area of the joint which is under the greatest mechanical load.
Consequently, it is subjected to very concentrated, intensely deforming weight-bearing

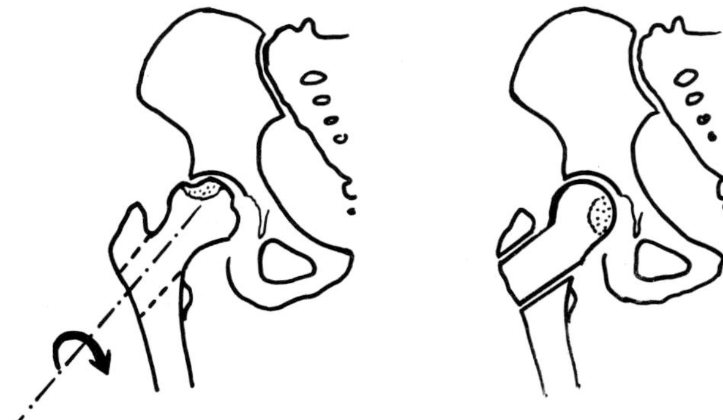

Fig. 7. Schematic representation of intertrochanteric double osteotomy with rotation of the
femoral neck on its longitudinal axis. The necrotic focus of the femoral head is rotated out of the
cranial segment of the joint into the anterocaudal joint area

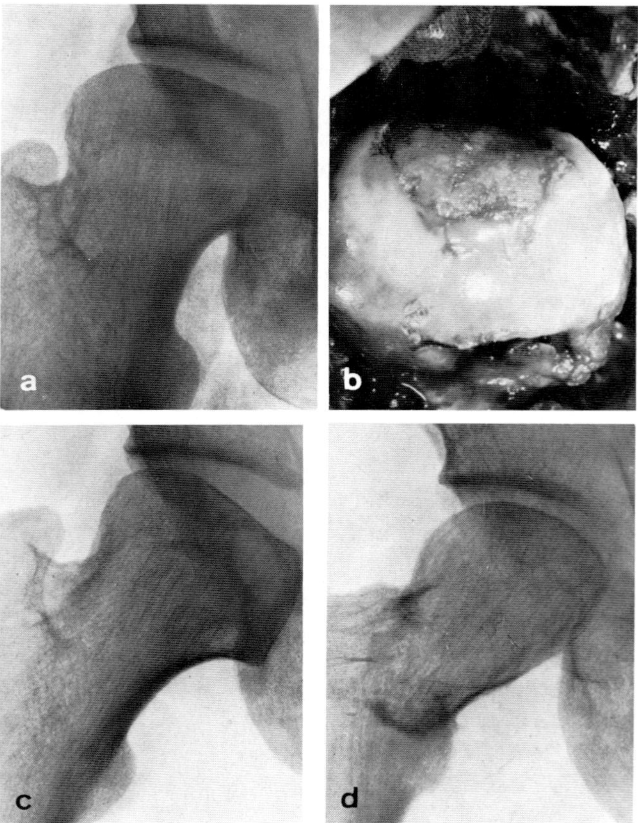

Fig. 8. a, b Femoral head necrosis in a 22-year-old girl with flattening of the cranial segment of the femoral head. **c** On internal rotation and abduction, congruency is lost between the deformed femoral head and the acetabulum. **d** Congruency of the articular surfaces after derotation, varisation and rotation of the femoral neck on its longitudinal axis condition 18 months after operation (Wagner 1967)

forces. When the leg is in neutral position, the usually sharp-edged anterolateral margin of the collapsed articular surface area lies opposite the anterosuperior acetabular margin (Fig. 9). When the hip joint is flexed even a few degrees, either the limbus is pinched between the edge of the femoral head defect and the acetabular margin, or the articular ridge of the femoral head is forced under the acetabular margin by a step-like motion mechanism. Both phenomena cause chronic painful irritation of the joint. Intertrochanteric osteotomy eliminates this motion anomaly by transferring the articular ridge of the femoral head away from the acetabular margin. This creates unimpeded motion, which is enhanced if a simultaneous valgus correction is performed.

Collapse of the necrotic segment of the femoral head also severely damages joint congruency, which can also be corrected by intertrochanteric osteotomy. The superior segment of the femoral head, which assumes a more cylindrical shape due to the collapse of the articular surface, is pressed against the spherical surface of the acetabulum at the cranial aspect of the joint, that area so important for joint mechanics. Stability of joint

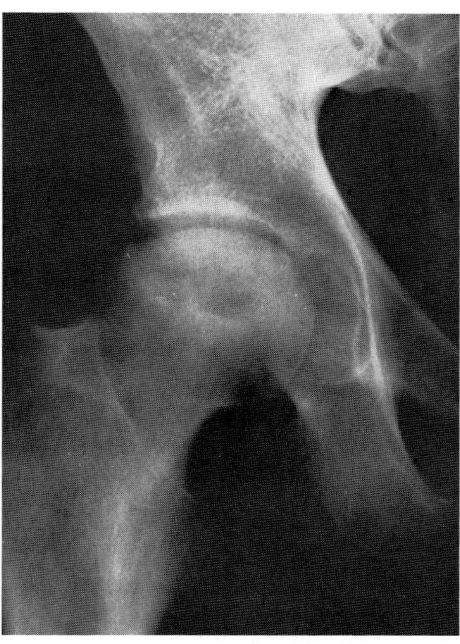

Fig. 9. Idiopathic necrosis of the femoral head with collapse of the articular surface into the necrotic segment. An articular ridge has formed on the lateral margin of the femoral head facing the acetabular rim and acts as a blocking structure

congruency is lost due to divergence in the curves of the acetabulum and of the femoral head. This situation is aggravated by the fact that, due to the joint surface impression, the femoral head drifts craniolaterally and leaves the center of the acetabulum. This results in loss of joint contact at the medial and inferior contact areas (Fig. 17). Intertrochanteric flexion-valgus osteotomy corrects this problem too and restores joint congruency. With this operation, the cylindrico-eliptical portion of the femoral head is moved away from the joint, and the spherical posteromedial area of the femoral head is brought into contact with the spherical articular surface of the acetabulum. Joint congruency is thus regained. In addition, optimal medial load transmission in the hip joint is obtained.

The valgus component of intertrochanteric osteotomy has further significance. When a flexion osteotomy is performed with the base of the wedge in a totally anterior position, physiological anteversion of the femoral neck is converted into a varus component which compromises medial load transmission in the joint, relaxes the pelvitrochanteric muscles, shortens the leg, and makes future joint replacement more difficult. These disadvantages may be avoided by additional valgus correction in which the base of the wedge is located anterolaterally. Valgus correction nevertheless results in lengthening of the leg, which increases joint pressure via increased tension in the soft tissue, particularly in the adductors. The lengthening effect can be avoided by resecting an equivalent bone segment at the site of the osteotomy. The necessary limb length measurement can be easily and exactly obtained by using an image intensifier. With the leg parallel to the table, the articular spaces of the hip and knee joints are projected into the *central ray* of the image intensifier, and a mark is made on the skin over the respective joint space. The distance between the two marks corresponds to the length of the femur. After femoral neck correction, the length is measured again in the same way before osteosynthesis is completed. The increase in length measured in this way corresponds with the required bone resection.

Finally, it should be borne in mind that when a flexion osteotomy is performed, the physiologic valgus position of the femoral neck is partly converted into anteversion, which can affect the rotational position of the leg. Therefore, care should be taken to ensure that internal rotation of at least 15° is still possible before the osteotomy is completed.

AO right-angle plates with a blade length of 45–55 mm have proven their worth for osteotomy stabilization. In cases of simultaneous valgus correction, where lateral displacement of the distal fragment is desirable, condylar plates may be used to bring the fragments in line at the lateral surface of the femur. Moreover, the condylar plate guarantees particularly good stability, since it allows additional fixation of 1–2 screws in the proximal fragment. In all intertrochanteric osteotomies, but particularly in valgus osteotomies, stability is considerably improved by firmly interwoven tension band sutures between the reinserted tendon origin of the vastus lateralis and the tendon of the glutaeus medius.

Indications for intertrochanteric osteotomy are limited by the extent of the necrotic focus. Careful radiologic examinations are required to determine focal size exactly. Standard AP and lateral projections provide a very good general survey. Observing motion on the image intensifier provides insight into sequential motion of the deformed articular surface and of congruency in diverse corrective positions. It also permits radiographs that pinpoint the largest focal diameter to be obtained. Valuable information on the condition of the articular surface can also be provided by lateral radiographs with the hip in different degrees of flexion and by angling the tube craniodorsally on the extended hip joint, as recommended by Schneider (1979). As a rule, a greater extent of the necrotic focus is revealed by lateral views than by AP radiographs. Focal size is measured in both planes by the angle between radii that emanate from the center of the femoral head and border on the focal margins. The total angle of the values obtained from each plane has proved valuable for practical assessment. Intertrochanteric osteotomy experience has shown that the critical limit for an osteotomy is total angle of 200°, i.e., focal sizes greater than 200° are too large for an osteotomy, and satisfactory results cannot be expected.

Careful clinical and radiologic analysis is required in the treatment of idiopathic necrosis of the femoral head by intertrochanteric flexion-valgus osteotomy, but the magnitude of the operation is relatively small. Weight-bearing can be permitted a few months after surgery. Since the femoral head is preserved, future alternative methods of treatment are still possible. After intertrochanteric osteotomy, articular pain almost always subsides immediately. The overwhelming majority of patients experience only minor discomfort and are able to withstand weight-bearing forces for a long time. On the other hand, even in pain-free hips reossification of the necrotic area develops only very slowly. Occasionally, a second intertrochanteric osteotomy can be performed at a later date on the same hip if femoral head deformity causing arthrosis deformans occurs in the future (Fig. 10).

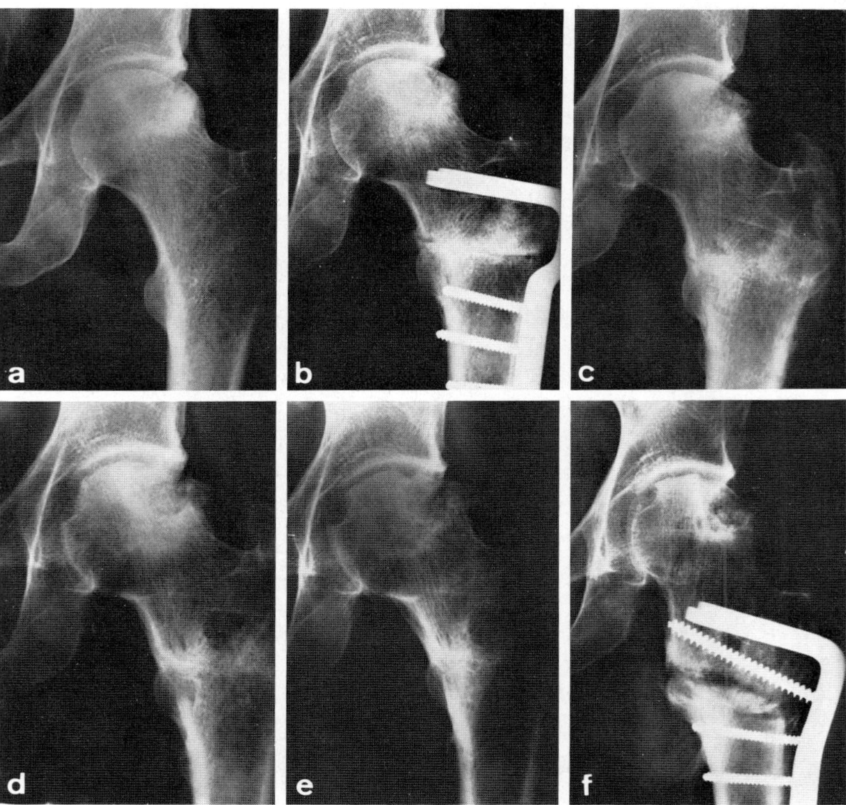

Fig. 10. a Idiopathic necrosis of the femoral head in 41-year-old man with a large necrotic focus and marked articular ridge formation. **b** Eight weeks after intertrochanteric flexion-valgus osteotomy with good opening of the lateral portion of the joint space and removal of the articular surface ridge from the lateral edge of the acetabular roof. **c** One year after osteotomy. **d** Three years after intertrochanteric osteotomy. Solid bone structure is present in the painfree joint, but there is initial osteophyte formation at the lateral edge of the femoral head. **e** Eight years after intertrochanteric osteotomy. Narrowing of the radiographic joint space, cylindric deformation of the craniolateral segment of the femoral head. Complaints after walking long distances and with abduction. **f** A second valgus osteotomy opens the lateral joint space and removes the lateral projections of the femoral head from its position at the cranial-acetabular margin

Total Joint Replacement

Total endoprosthetic hip replacement is often required when the extent of large necrotic foci exceeds the critical limit within which intertrochanteric osteotomy may be performed. Except for the necrotic focus, there is usually very good bone quality. Therefore, conditions for total joint replacement would be particularly favorable if the young age of the patient and frequent bilateral involvement of the hip joint did not necessitate restraint. As is well-known, temptation to perform a total joint replacement is great because pain and functional impairment are immediately eliminated and the patient regains normal physical well-being after only a few weeks. Nevertheless, complications caused by implant loosening are indeed very discouraging.

Joint Resurfacing

During recent years, resurfacing of the hip joint has been a good compromise to hip joint replacement in cases of idiopathic femoral head necrosis (Wagner 1978a, 1979). This method allows better alternatives after implant loosening, since only the articular surfaces of the femoral head and acetabulum are replaced by hemispherical cup implants, while the femoral head and neck is preserved. This is particularly important for young patients.

As yet, there has been very little experience with resurfacing in cases of idiopathic femoral head necrosis. We began to use this procedure in April 1976 for such conditions. Initially we employed it very sparingly as we were afraid of an increased risk of loosening due to bone necrosis of the femoral head. This fear has not yet been substantiated. On the contrary, no loosening of the implant has occurred so far in cases of idiopathic femoral head necrosis. Rather, observations imply that in young patients idiopathic necrosis of the femoral head is a particularly good indication for resurfacing. This is probably due to the particularly good state of the bone tissue surrounding the necrotic focus, which is characterized by mechanical stability and hyperemia.

Observations made during prosthetic replacement for genuine coxarthrosis can also provide information on this matter. One hip joint revision was performed 5 years and 3 months after resurfacing, due to discomfort from scar tissue with heterotopic ossification. The opportunity was used to replace implants which were still stable but required improvement of their position. The femoral component was pulled from the cement bed, and the intact layer of cement was smashed into several pieces by using an osteotome and was then removed. Relatively severe bone atrophy was revealed in the center of the femoral head, whereas peripheral layers of bone in continuation with the cortex of the femoral neck resembled solid ivory over the entire circumference of the femoral head. This seems to show that resurfacing does not distribute loading forces evenly over the entire surface of the bone below the femoral component, as we previously assumed. The center of the femoral head is obviously subjected to very slight stress, while the main loading forces are transferred to the superficial layers of the femoral head and neck via the margins of the implant. However, these superficial layers of bone, which are obviously so crucial, are in particularly good condition in idiopathic femoral head necrosis, even when large foci with marked collapse of the articular surface are present. On the contrary, according to this observation, the femoral head defect, which is filled with spongiosa grafts after removal of the necrotic tissue, does not play a significant role in sustaining loading forces, which may help to explain the success of our results so far.

Therefore, during resurfacing the lateral weight-bearing border of the femoral head must be preserved and completely covered by the femoral component (Figs. 11, 12). This not only applies to cases of idiopathic necrosis of the femoral head, but is a fundamental principle of resurfacing implantation. In the presence of extensive subtotal necrosis of the femoral head, which requires shortening of the femoral neck and possibly displacement of the greater trochanter, the lateral cortex of the femoral neck must be preserved and covered by the lateral edge of the femoral component. This detail has not been stated as strongly in previous publications and is therefore particularly emphasized here.

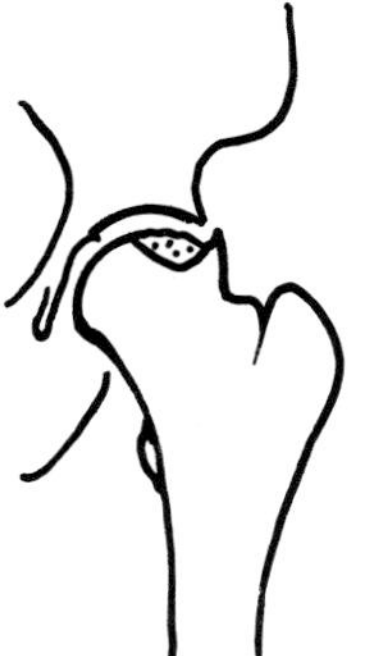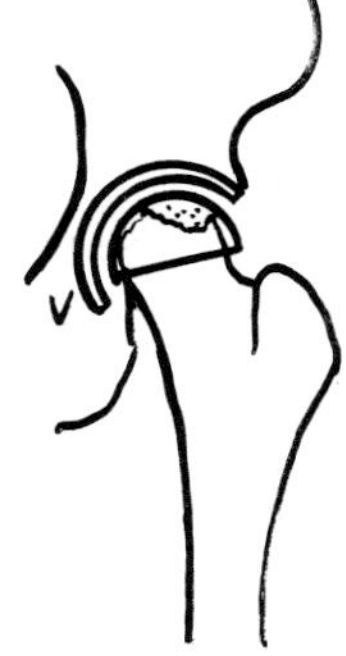

Fig. 11. Schematic representation of the position of a resurfacing prosthesis for idiopathic necrosis of the femoral head. The lateral edge of the femoral head is preserved and covered by the femoral component; if necessary, excess bone tissue must be removed from medial and ventral portions of the head

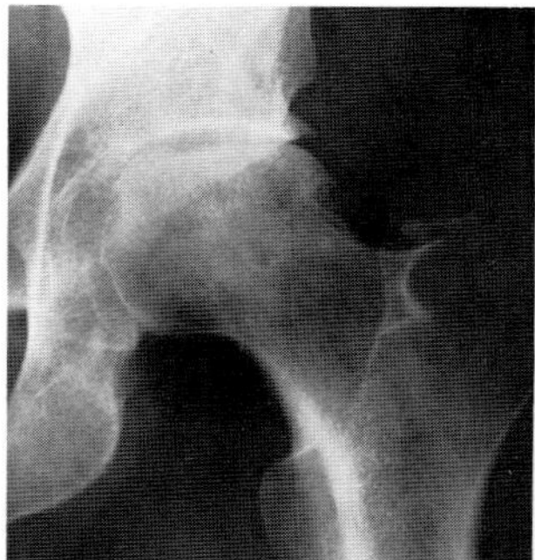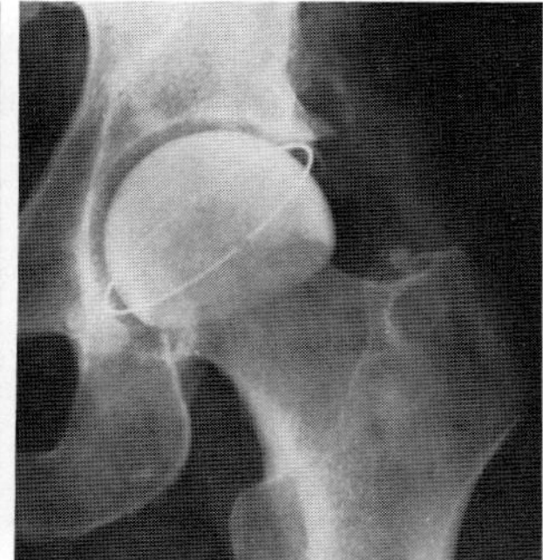

Fig. 12. Example of resurfacing prosthesis fitting for idiopathic necrosis of the femoral head. The lateral margin of the femoral head is preserved and covered by a ceramic femoral component

However, despite all its advantages, resurfacing must still be regarded at present as a compromise or temporary solution. It should only be used on the basis of very critical indications. Restraint is strongly recommended by the mere fact that the follow-up period for this method of treatment is only 6 years, and only a little more than 4.5 years in cases of idiopathic necrosis of the femoral head. According to present knowledge, resurfacing is only indicated in cases in which the patient's suffering compels operative intervention, joint-preserving osteotomies are no longer possible, and strong reservations exist against arthrodesis or total joint replacement.

When considering indications for resurfacing, it must be remembered that a well-fitted total joint replacement is better for the patient than a poorly fitted resurfacing prosthesis. It is technically far more difficult to correctly implant a resurfacing prosthesis than a total prosthesis. Technical errors, which are tolerated for years by a total joint replacement, will result in early loosening of the resurfacing prosthesis due to the small surface area for anchorage. It is unfortunate that not all technical errors, for example, the mishandling of bone cement, are detectable by radiography, and that these errors cannot always be analyzed even by a second operation. Due to the degree of technical difficulty, resurfacing will not become an "everyman's procedure." Good results will always depend on the quality of the experienced hip surgeon. In recent years we have noted with anxiety that many surgeons have turned to resurfacing without knowing the proper technique of this operation or possible alternative methods to hip surgery. This should be avoided since it is harmful for the patient and detracts from the success of the method.

Results

Since 1967, 184 hip joints have been treated operatively at our hospital for idiopathic necrosis of the femoral head (Table 1). Intertrochanteric osteotomy was performed on the largest group of patients, that is, on 108 hip joints. Total joint replacement was carried out on 47 hips and a resurfacing procedure on 13 hip joints. Subchondral spongiosa plasty was performed on ten hip joints and arthrodesis on six hip joints.

Table 1. Hip joints operated since 1967 for idiopathic necrosis of the femoral head

Intertrochanteric osteotomy	108 hips
Total prosthesis	47 hips
Resurfacing prosthesis	13 hips
Subchondral spongiosa plasty	10 hips
Arthrodesis	6 hips
Total	184 hips

A comparison of these figures does not reveal the change in therapy. The change is characterized by the facts that the number of patients with idiopathic femoral head necrosis has steadily increased over the years and that subchondral spongiosa plasty has been practically discontinued in favor of intertrochanteric osteotomy. In recent years, more emphasis has been placed on the valgus component of intertrochanteric flexion osteotomy. Total joint replacement has decreased in the past 4 years in favor of resurfacing. Hip arthrodesis has been, and still is, used only in exceptional circumstances.

Results of Intertrochanteric Osteotomy

The following analysis of our results with intertrochanteric osteotomy was carried out on a group of patients who were operated on between January 1968 and December 1978. These patients received standardized treatment, and all fundamental criteria were comparable. Patients who were operated on before 1968 are not included, since prior to that date operative technique was not standardized and the number of patients was small. Similarly, the study does not include patients who were operated on after 1978, since the postoperative follow-up period is too short.

In the period from 1968 to 1978, 83 intertrochanteric osteotomies were performed in 71 patients (Table 2). Bilateral involvement occurred in 19 patients, and bilateral osteotomies were performed in 12 of these in a second operation. The number of males far exceeded the number of females (66 to 5). Of the 83 joints, 69 have been recently

Table 2. Eighty-three intertrochanteric flexion osteotomies from 1968–78

71 patients	66 men
	5 women
Bilateral involvement	19 patients
Bilateral osteotomy	12 patients

Table 3. Age of the patients in years at the time of intertrochanteric osteotomy

25	31	33	36	38	41	43	49	59
25	31	33	36	38	41	44	50	61
27	31	33	36	38	41	44	51	65
28	31	33	36	38	41	44	51	
29	31	33	36	38	42	47	52	
29	32	35	36	39	42	47	53	
29	32	35	36	39	42	47	56	
29	32	35	37	40	42	48	57	
30	32	35	37	40	42	48	57	
30	33	35	38	41	43	48	58	

Average age 39.5 years

reexamined. Three patients had died, and reexaminations of the remaining patients had been performed quite some time ago. At the time of surgery, the average age of the patients was 39.5 years (Table 3). The youngest patient was 25 years old, the oldest 65 years old. Eight patients were under 30 years, 47 patients under 40, and 71 patients under 50.

Before being seen at our hospital for the first time, the patients had experienced pain for 2–48 months, with an average of 11.5 months. Twelve patients had not received previous medical treatment, while 25 patients had received conservative treatment over a long period. In three cases, operative treatment had been performed in a different hospital. At the beginning of treatment, all patients complained of moderate to severe pain.

Predisposing associated diseases or metabolic disorders were present in at least 29 patients (Table 4). Hyperuricemia was noted in 14 patients, histological evidence of liver parenchyma damage was found in four patients, hyperlipidemia was present in one patient and diabetes mellitus was manifested in two patients. Pain occurred immediately after pregnancy in one patient. Six patients admitted to chronic alcohol abuse, but ambiguous figures have to be expected in regard to this problem.

Table 4. Predisposing illnesses or metabolic disorders

Hyperuricemia	14 patients
Liver parenchyma damage	4 patients
Diabetes mellitus	2 patients
Hyperlipidemia	1 patient
Pregnancy	1 patient
Alcoholism	6 (?) patients

Table 5. Condition of hip joints prior to surgery

Intact spherical shape of the femoral head	11 hip joints
Flattening of the focal surface	15 hip joints
Ridge formation on the focal margin	14 hip joints
Extensive collaspe of the articular surface	43 hip joints
Lateralization of the femoral head	15 hip joints
Arthrosis of the femoral head	30 hip joints
Arthrosis of the acetabulum	13 hip joints

During preoperative planning, the condition of the articular surface of the femoral head was very carefully analyzed, and focal size was determined radiologically, as already described (Table 5). The spherical shape of the femoral head was preserved in 11 joints, as seen in the radiographs. Advanced changes of the articular surface were noted in a large number of hip joints, matching the long, painful course of the disease prior to therapy. Flattening of the articular surface in the focal area had occurred in 15 hip joints, ridges in the articular surface were already present in 14 cases, and widespread collapse of the articular surface has occurred in 43 cases. Lateralization had already taken place in 15 femoral heads. This was accompanied by a buildup of bony tissue in the acetabular floor. These changes are almost exclusively found when the disease has been present for more than a year. Reactive arthrotic changes were evident in 30 femoral heads and in 13 acetabula.

The long average time span of almost a year between the onset of pain and the beginning of clinical treatment is noteworthy. Operative treatment was immediately initiated in all patients since not only demarcation of necrotic foci had already occurred, but the best time to operate had also been exceeded for most patients, as extensive collapse of the articular surface and arthrotic changes were already present in the hip joints. When universal damage of the hip joint with reactive arthrotic changes has occurred, less success has to be expected after an osteotomy than if no secondary changes are present at the time of surgery.

The angle of flexion required for correction was almost exclusively between 30° and 40°. Flexion up to 60° was only required in a few specific cases. Flexion correction was combined with a valgus correction of 15–25° in 70 of the 83 osteotomies.

Varus correction of the femoral neck is theoretically justified when a necrotic focus is located quite far medially and abuts against a large healthy section of the lateral articular surface. This usually occurs only in partial posttraumatic necrosis of the femoral head and never in idiopathic necrosis. Consequently, we have observed that the worst results were obtained from the few varus corrections performed on our patients.

The adverse effect of varus positioning lies in the fact that it counteracts turning the necrotic area away from the acetabular margin, which flexion osteotomy attempts to achieve. Moreover, cranial shift of the greater trochanter weakens the pelvitrochanteric muscles and ultimately makes future prosthetic joint replacement more difficult.

Postoperatively, partial weight was born on the operated limb by using two forearm crutches for 3 months. Delayed bony union, which has been described as typical for cases of idiopathic femoral head necrosis, could not be found. As a rule, bony union occurred 3 months after osteotomy. Partial weight-bearing by using forearm crutches over even a longer period of time aids convalescence and structural recovery of the damaged joint.

Bony union took 4–6 months in only 6 of the 83 cases. One patient in this group loosened the osteosynthesis by full weight-bearing, and the angle plate had to be recompressed. One infection occurred at the osteotomy site, but healing took place after the metallic implant had been removed. In the four other cases, radiographs taken immediately after the operation showed insufficient medial support of the fragment.

After the operation, there was considerable correlation between discomfort and objective findings. Immediate pain relief, which occurred after osteotomy, was particularly impressive. Regression of discomfort was prolonged in only a few cases. During the first follow-up examination 8 weeks after the operation, only four patients complained of substantial hip pain. Subsequently these four patients never became painfree.

Several patients experienced discomfort in the "hip area" after painfree periods of many years. The discomfort did not originate in the hip joint but was caused by tendinoses in the periarticular region. It responded well to local symptomatic therapy.

The latest follow-up examination revealed discomfort in only 10 of the 69 hip joints. Valuable conclusions may be drawn by analyzing these cases. Unsatisfactory regression of discomfort can be explained by an excessively large necrotic focus, advanced preoperative arthrotic changes of the hip joint, and varus position of the femoral neck after the operation. Only 4 of the 69 joints reexamined were never free of pain after the operation. Two of these cases displayed subtotal necrosis with an total angle of 280° in the two planes. A varization of 25° had been performed in addition to flexion osteotomy in one of these joints. A varisation of 30° without flexion osteotomy had been done in the third case. The fourth patient has complained of pain since the operation. His discomfort cannot be explained as his musculature is equally well-developed bilaterally, and very good motion with a radiologically wide joint space is present 4 years after the osteotomy.

After a painfree period of 2–3 years, painful impairment of hip joint function recurred in three patients. Initially, subtotal necrosis was present in two of these patients. In one of these two patients, total joint replacement was carried out 4 years after the osteotomy. In the third patient, radiographs showed long-lasting bone atrophy and progressive functional deterioration after varus correction.

In one case, pain recurred 4 years after a combined flexion-varus osteotomy. Another very obese patient was free of pain for only a year. Slight discomfort recurred in another patient 9 years after the osteotomy. His preoperative radiologic findings consisted of a necrotic focus with an total angle of 210°, extensive collapse of the femoral head, and arthrotic changes.

A repeat intertrochanteric valgus osteotomy was performed in another patient who, 8 years after the osteotomy, finally developed painful arthrotic changes on weight-bearing and an oval deformity of the femoral head (Fig. 10).

Since we expected that results of intertrochanteric osteotomy would depend largely on the size of the necrotic focus, we compared groups of hip joints with approximately equal focal size. In one group of 24 painfree hip joints with very good clinical and radiologic results, the necrosis angle was between 50° and 90° on the AP view and between 60° and 100° on the lateral view. Without exception, the total necrosis on both planes remained below 200°. The articular surface in all these cases was judged to be intact or only slightly flattened (Figs. 13, 14).

A necrotic angle of 90°–100° was revealed by AP radiograph and of 100°–130° by lateral

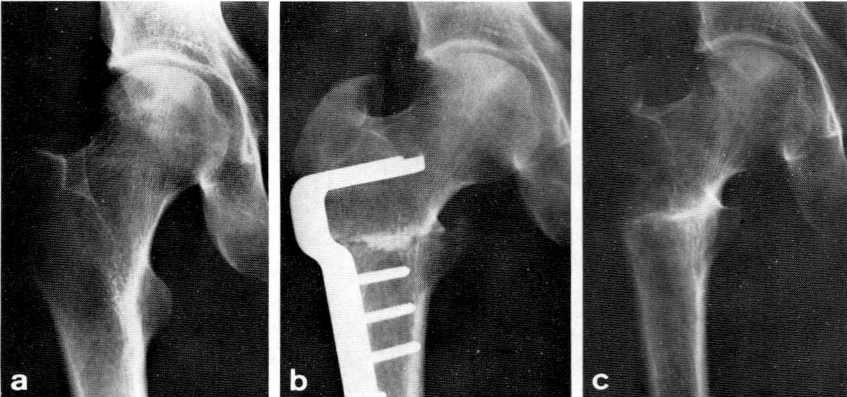

Fig. 13. a Idiopathic necrosis of the femoral head in a 42-year-old man (the same patient as in Fig. 10). **b** Three months after intertrochanteric valgus-flexion osteotomy. **c** Seven years after osteotomy: the necrotic focus was smaller than on the opposite side, and no reactive changes had yet occurred (see Fig. 10). Seven years after the osteotomy, a well-maintained joint space and improved bone structure in the focal area were present and corresponded to normal pain-free function

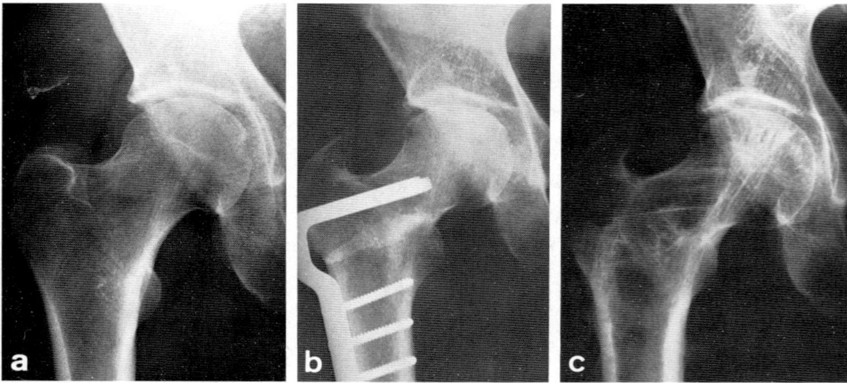

Fig. 14. Idiopathic necrosis of the femoral head in a 38-year-old man. **a** Initial radiologic findings show favorable focal size, no secondary arthrotic changes, and no articular surface deformity. **b** Six months after intertrochanteric flexion-valgus osteotomy. **c** Five years after the operation with sound radiologic joint space and normal painfree function

radiograph in a group of 30 painfree hip joints. Initial findings revealed extensive collapse of the femoral head, and in 14 cases the onset of arthrotic changes. The average value of the total necrosis angle was 220°. Radiologic findings deteriorated over the years in this group. In contrast to the first group, there has been a gradual increase of articular surface deformity and of arthrotic changes in this group (Figs. 15, 16).

In the group where hip joint pain persisted or recurred, there were six cases with subtotal necrotic foci, in which the total necrosis angle in both planes was between 230° and 280°. This obviously exceeds the limit within which intertrochanteric osteotomy may be successfully performed. The narrow healthy remaining segment of the femoral head is no longer able to maintain stable joint congruency with the acetabulum. Instability and

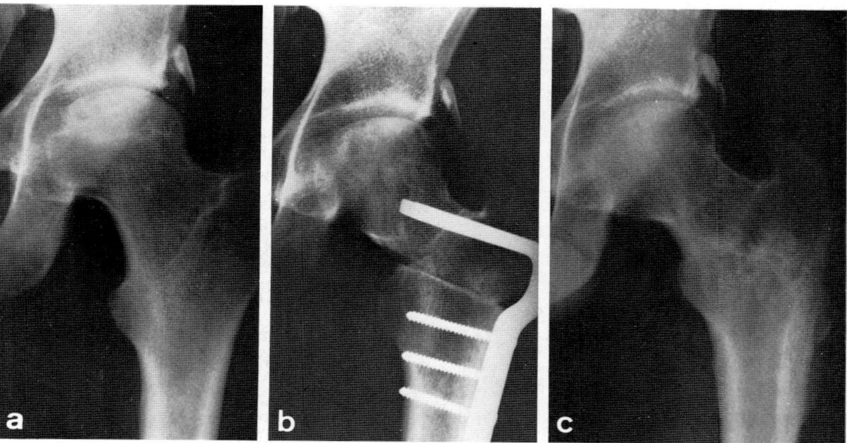

Fig. 15. a Extensive idiopathic necrosis of the femoral head in a 27-year-old man. b Six weeks after intertrochanteric flexion-valgus osteotomy. c Six years after osteotomy. Despite painfree function and a wide radiologic joint space, slight collapse of the articular surface is present due to the large size of the focus

large defects in the articular surface cause synovial irritation, which in turn gradually destroys the still intact sections of the acetabular surface and promotes the advance of arthrosis deformans (Figs. 17, 18).

It is obvious that a close connection exists between focal size and arthrotic changes present prior to the osteotomy on the one hand and the postoperative condition of the hip joint on the other. Thus, in 11 cases where an intact articular surface and a small focal site were noted as initial findings and which remained unchanged up to the end of the postoperative follow-up period, a radiologically wide joint space was evident in all hip joints, and no deformity of the articular surface developed in nine of these hips. Only the two remaining femoral heads showed a slight indentation at the focal area. Complete reossification of the necrotic focus occurred in six of these cases. Therefore, intertrochanteric osteotomy can effectively protect the necrotic area from deformity until revitalization takes place in a fair number of these early cases.

When initial findings reveal larger sizes of articular surface defects, then steady progression of the articular surface deformity and arthrotic reactions during the course of the observation period will occur. After focal collapse has transpired, intertrochanteric osteotomy can still remove the ridge on the articular surface of the femoral head from direct contact with the acetabular margin. However, slight chronic synovial irritation and the gradual advance of joint deterioration cannot be completely avoided. Radiologically, an amazingly wide cranial joint space persists for a long time, despite anatomical changes in the articular surface. However, in several cases, there was a marked discrepancy between the patient's continued relief from pain and clearly visible signs of deterioration in the radiograph.

Revitalization and reossification of the necrotic focus depend, as already stated, on focal size and the initial condition of the articular surface. Complete bony restoration occurred within 2–3 years in 6 of the 11 hip joints which belonged to the group demon-

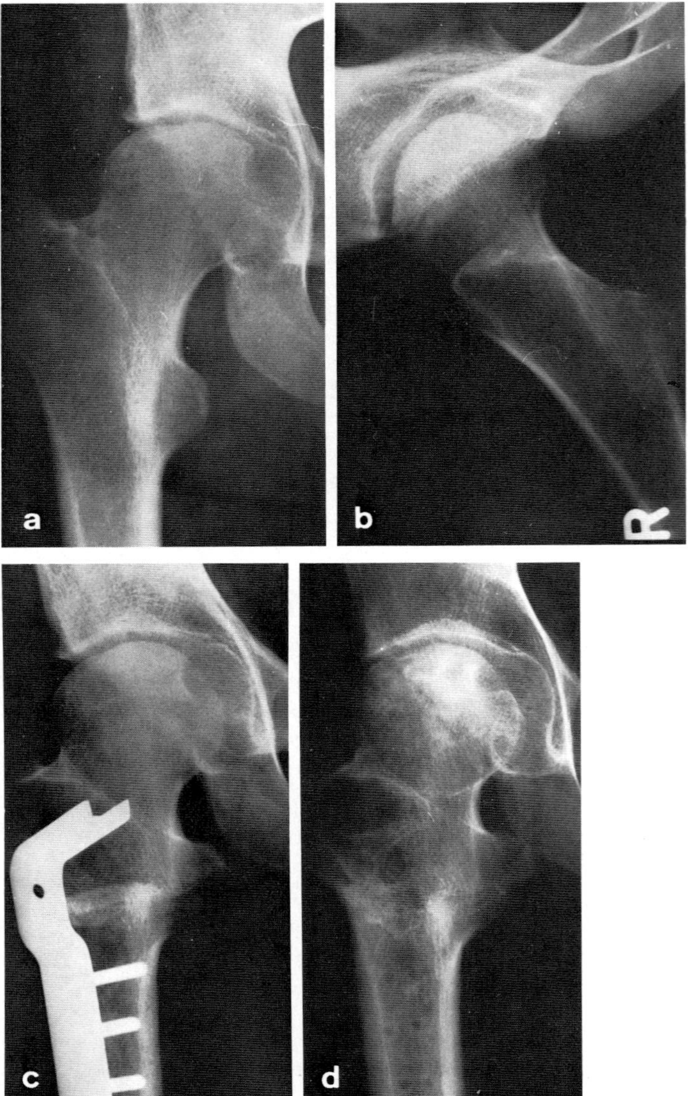

Fig. 16.a, b Extensive idiopathic necrosis of the femoral head in a 25-year-old man. **c** Six weeks after intertrochanteric flexion-valgus osteotomy with a marked valgus component. **d** Four years after osteotomy, good painfree function is present. Configuration of the trajectorial bone structure of the femoral head and acetabular roof reveal extensive medial transference of load transmission, yet there is slight secondary collapse of the articular surface in the craniolateral section of the femoral head

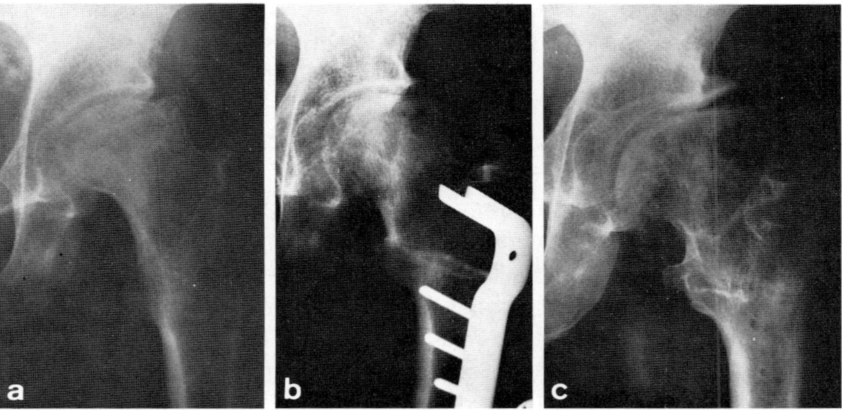

Fig. 17. a Extensive idiopathic necrosis of the femoral head with major collapse of the articular surface but wide radiological joint space in a 33-year-old man. **b** Eight weeks after intertrochanteric flexion-valgus osteotomy with good medialization of the femoral head and widening of the lateral joint space. **c** Twelve years after intertrochanteric osteotomy, marked secondary arthrotic deformities of the articular surface of the femoral head and acetabulum are present. The slight complaints of discomfort stated by the patient are explained by the wide joint space and favorable configuration of the medial segment

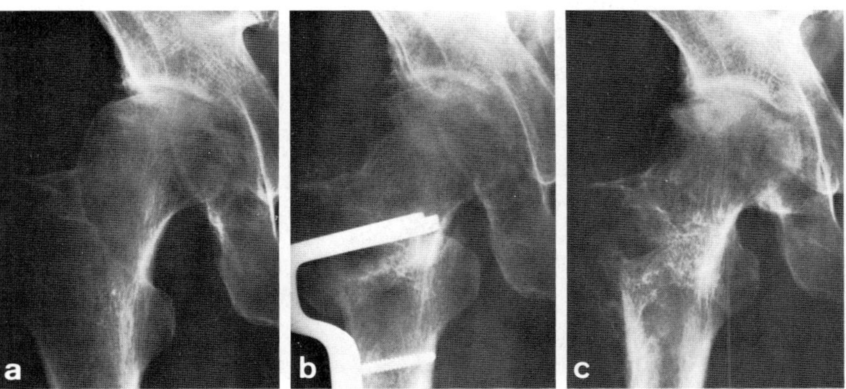

Fig. 18.a Extensive idiopathic necrosis of the femoral head in a 56-year-old man with articular surface deformity and advance secondary arthrotic changes. **b** Eight weeks after intertrochanteric flexion-valgus osteotomy with insufficient improvement in congruency of the joint space. **c** Four years after osteotomy, renewed increase in pain with reduced motion and marked deformity and narrowing of the joint space

strating intact spherical articular surfaces. Bony restoration occurred only twice in the 15 hip joints with flattened articular surfaces. There was not one example of *complete* reossification in 57 hip joints, where ridges had formed on the margin of the focus or where extensive collapse has occurred. Depending on the time interval after osteotomy, necrotic foci showed bony reconstitution in 25%–50%. Therefore, in such initial findings, complete revitalization of the necrotic areas should not be expected for 5 years or more after osteotomy.

Mobility of the hip joint after intertrochanteric osteotomy essentially depends on the preoperative condition of the joint. In necrotic areas where the total necrosis angle lies within the range favoring intertrochanteric osteotomy, mobility can be preserved for a long time, and it is often even improved. Gradual reduction in mobility usually occurs over the course of time if the total necrosis angle reaches borderline values or if it exceeds the limit.

At the end of the follow-up period, 30 hip joints showed improvement in hinge motion of 5°–40°, with an average of 25°. Without exception, these were patients who were pain-free and who had radiologically a wide joint space. Compared to preoperative findings, there was no change in the range of motion of 25 hip joints.

In 14 hip joints, hinge motion had decreased by 10°–40°. Extension was limited by 10°–15° in five of these patients. All of the ten painful hip joints mentioned above belonged to this group. The value of routine detachment of the ventral hip joint capsule and consequent postoperative therapeutic positioning and exercises is confirmed by the fact that extension limitation occurs relatively rarely.

In all 30 hip joints of the first group, abduction was unchanged, or sometimes it even showed definite improvement. In 16 other hip joints, abduction was generally slightly reduced, mostly after varisation, and in 24 hip joints with a marked valgus component, adduction was reduced by 5°–20° without producing an abduction contracture.

Early on in our series, internal rotation was severely reduced. This problem has been solved since we aim for an internal rotation component of at least 15° intraoperatively. The group of 15 hip joints with slightly reduced external rotation corresponds with that having restricted motion in all directions. It also includes all patients with painful joints.

Additional operations are generally not required after intertrochanteric flexion-valgus osteotomy with correction of limb-length discrepancy. In the group of patients studied, trochanteric transposition was required in two cases due to a high-riding trochanter with insufficiency of the pelvitrochanteric musculature after varus osteotomy. In one case, a modified pelvic osteotomy was performed to improve coverage of the femoral head. Evacuation of a wound hematoma was required once. If performed earlier, the resulting wound infection could probably have been avoided.

There were no serious complications such as proven pulmonary emobilisations or deaths.

Results of Hip Joint Resurfacing

Patients who were treated by resurfacing for avascular necrosis of the femoral head represent an extraordinarily heterogenous group. Because at first we had no experience with replacement of the articular surface in cases of femoral head necrosis and feared that a surface prosthesis would not be well tolerated, we used the resurfacing procedure only in particularly problematic conditions where, in our opinion, no other legitimate alternative was available.

Since April 1976, 13 hip joints have undergone resurfacing for ischemic necrosis. This involved 11 patients, 2 of whom had bilateral involvement. Patients were between ages 30 and 50, with an average of 38.5 years (Table 6). There was a far greater ratio of males to

Table 6. Age at time of resurfacing

30 years	35 years	46 years
30 years	38 years	46 years
30 years	38 years	50 years
35 years	43 years	
35 years	44 years	

Average age 38.5 years

females, namely 9 to 4. It should be noted that there were only two women in the group of 11 patients, and both had bilateral involvement. One woman was an alcoholic, the other had received long-term cortisone treatment after a kidney transplantation.

So-called idiopathic necrosis of the femoral head was present in nine hip joints. A longer period of cortisone therapy had been necessary after renal transplants in two patients, one of whom had unilateral involvement, the other bilateral involvement. Femoral head necrosis caused by caisson disease was present in another patient.

Without exception, severe advanced conditions were found in all 13 hip joints. An impression of the condition of the hip joint was indirectly provided by the length of time pain had existed prior to the operation, which on an average was 38 months. Most of these patients had been previously told that their relatively young age prevented total hip joint replacement. Therefore they had received symptomatic conservative therapy. Three patients were no longer able to walk at the time of the operation (Figs. 19, 20).

A metallic femoral component was implanted in nine hip joints and a ceramic femoral component in four hip joints. A large resurfacing prosthesis with a femoral diameter of 50 mm was used on four occasions, an average-sized of 46 mm diameter was used seven times, and a small prosthesis with a 42 mm diameter was used twice. Postoperative follow-up revealed a particularly frequent tendency for heterotopic ossification. Marked heterotopic ossification was present in six hip joints (Fig. 21). There was no soft tissue

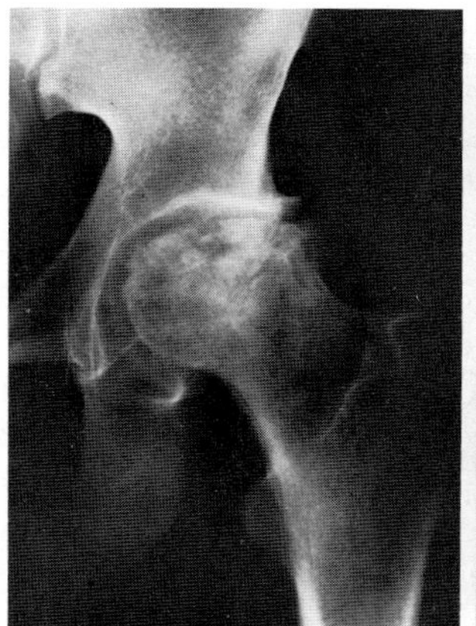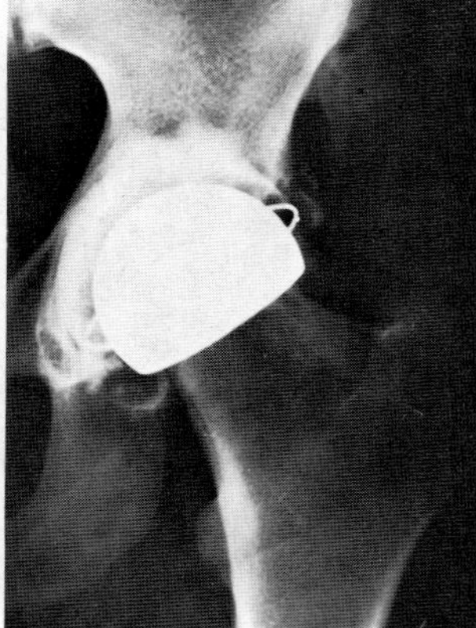

Fig. 19. Very extensive necrosis of the femoral head after kidney transplant in a 30-year-old woman (bilateral involvement). Three years after resurfacing, sound structural conditions are demonstrated by the radiograph

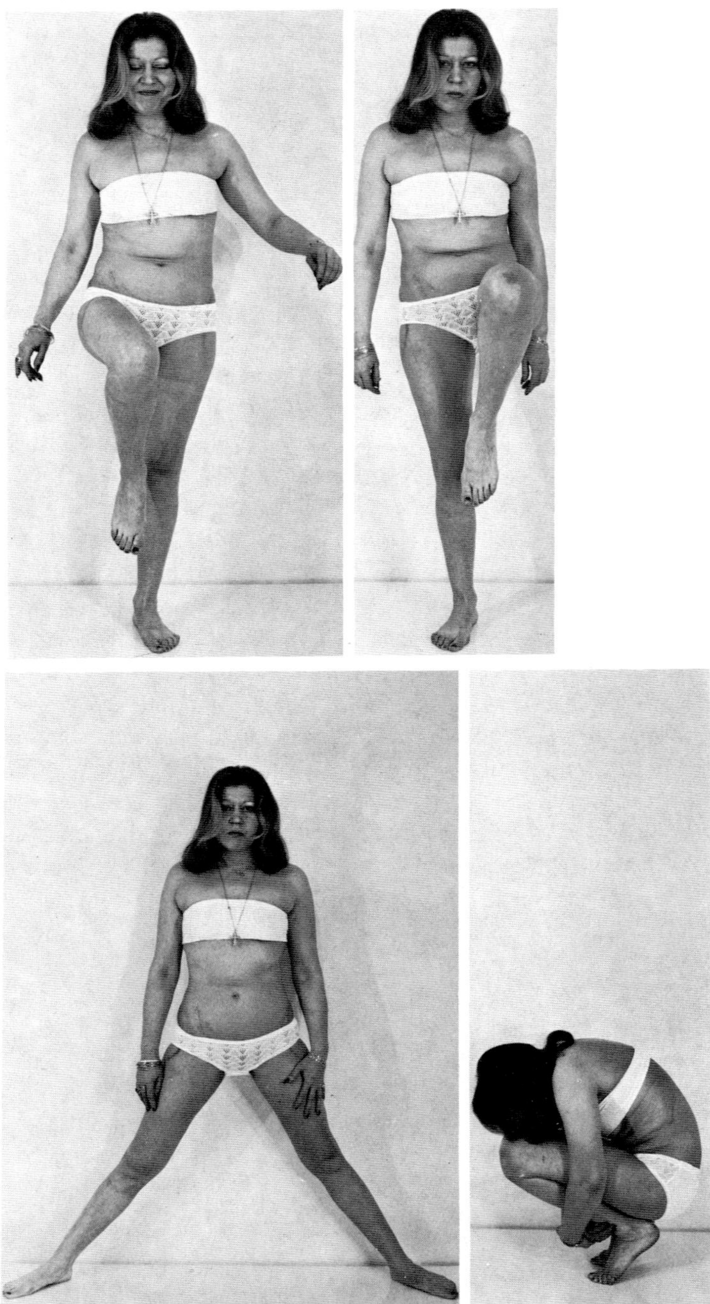

Fig. 20. The same patient as in Fig. 19 after bilateral resurfacing. Painfree normal function is present

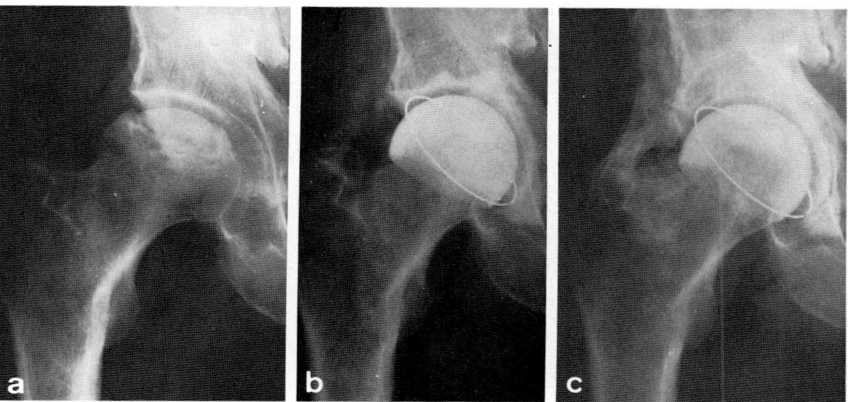

Fig. 21. a Extensive idiopathic necrosis of the femoral head in a 50-year-old man. **b** Four weeks after resurfacing. **c** Two years after resurfacing, marked periarticular ossification is present with reduced hinge motion but marked improvement in abduction and rotatory motion contrary to initial findings

ossification in seven hip joints. Nevertheless, periarticular ossification actually affected joint motion in only one hip joint, where hinge motion decreased from 100° to 60° while abduction in the same hip increased from 25° to 60° and rotatory motion increased from 15° to 35°.

On an average, all hip joints showed improved motion in all planes, i.e., hinge motion from 92° to 93°, abduction from 40° to 58°, and rotatory motion from 36° to 46°. The insignificant increase in average hinge motion is explained by the one case with heterotopic bone formation that resulted in severe loss of motion.

All operations were performed without complications. Immediate elimination of pain, which is typical of alloplastic joint replacement, was noted in all 13 hips. It was particularly impressive due to the severe preoperative changes. All hip joints were unweighted for 3 months by using two forearm crutches and protected for a further 3 months by using one forearm crutch. The postoperative observation period is more than 4 years in five hip joints, more than 3 years in four hip joints, more than 2 years in two hip joints, and more than 1 year in two hip joints.

No loosening of the resurfacing prosthesis occurred during the follow-up period. We even found rapid restoration and stabilization of the bone structure at the acetabulum and femoral neck with all prostheses. So far, according to these experiences, idiopathic necrosis of the femoral head is a good indication for joint resurfacing.

Summary

Intertrochanteric flexion-valgus-rotational osteotomy which preserves the joint is a important and efficient method to treat cases of idiopathic necrosis of the femoral head, which usually threatens younger patients by its rampant destruction of the joint and the frequent bilateral involvement, resulting in most severe impairment. Essentially, success of intertrochanteric osteotomy depends on the preoperative condition of the joint. The indication to perform an intertrochanteric osteotomy is limited by the site of the necrotic focus of the femoral head and by the degree of secondary arthrotic changes. Focal size can be successfully determined by the "total necrotic angle," i.e., the sum of the angles of the arc segments occupied by the necrotic focus on radiographs taken in two planes. The critical total necrotic angle for intertrochanteric osteotomy is 200°. Analysis of 83 intertrochanteric osteotomies with a follow-up period of up to more than 12 years shows that good long-term therapeutic results are to be expected when focal sizes are below this critical total angle. In cases of larger focal size, one has to make the decision if alloplastic joint replacement with its corresponding problems should be undertaken.

Experience with 13 hip joints over more than 4 years has shown that idiopathic necrosis of the femoral head is a good indication for joint resurfacing. Since the femoral head and neck are preserved, alternative methods of treatment are still possible in the future. Arthrodesis of the hip joint should only be considered on rare occasions for idiopathic necrosis of the femoral head.

References

Boettcher WG, Bonfiglio M, Hamilton HH, Sheets RF, Smith K (1970) Non-traumatic necrosis of the femoral head. J Bone Joint Surg [Am] 52:312

Eichler J (1974) Knochennekrosen bei Fettstoffwechselstörungen. Orthop Prax 10:758

Ficat P, Arlet J (1977) Ischémie et nécrose osseuses. Masson, Paris

Ganz R, Noesberger B (1978) Die posttraumatische Coxarthrose und ihre Behandlungsmöglichkeiten. Unfallheilkunde 81:238

Hungerford DS (1979) Bone marrow pressure, venography and core decompression in ischemic necrosis of the femoral head. In: The Hip. Mosby, St Louis, pp 218–238

Liebig K, Weseloh G (1977) Störung des Gelenkstoffwechsels bei der idiopatischen Hüftkopfnekrose. Z Orthop 115:477

Merle D'Aubigné R, Postel M, Mazabrand A, Massias P, Gueguen J (1965) Idiopathic necrosis of the femoral head in adults. J Bone Joint Surg [Br] 47:612

Müller ME (1971) Die hüftnahen Femurosteotomien. Thieme, Stuttgart

Patterson RJ, Bickel WH, Dahlin DC (1964) Idiopathic avascular necrosis of the head of the femur. J Bone Joint Surg [Am] 46:267

Pohl W (1971) Hüftkopfnekrosen bei Hyperlipidämie. Z Orthop 109:873

Schneider R (1979) Die intertrochantere Osteotomie bei Coxarthrose. Springer, Berlin Heidelberg New York

Sugioka Y (1973) Transtrochanteric anterior rotation osteotomy of the femoral head for avascular necrosis in adults. Cent Jpn J Orthop Traum Surg 16:574

Wagner H (1967) Ätiologie, Pathogenese, Klinik und Therapie der idiopatischen Hüftkopfnekrose. Verh Dtsch Orthop Ges 54:224

Wagner H (1972) Möglichkeiten und klinische Erfahrungen mit der Knorpeltransplantation. Z Orthop 110:705

Wagner H (1977) Prinzipien der Korrekturosteotomie am Bein. Orthopäde 6:145

Wagner H (1978a) Surface replacement arthroplasty of the hip. Clin Orthop 134:102

Wagner H (1978b) Beckenosteotomie bei der posttraumatischen Hüftkopfnekrose. Unfallheilkunde 81:188

Wagner H (1979) Die Schalenprothese des Hüftgelenkes-Oberflächenersatz als Gelenkerhaltung. Orthopäde 8:276

Zsernaviczky J, von Torklus D, Wilke H (1976) Aseptische Hüftkopfnekrose und Fettstoffwechselstörung Typ II nach Fredrickson. Z Orthop 114:100

Translation from the German: Wagner H, Zeiler G (1980) Idiopathische Hüftkopfnekrose. Orthopäde 9:290–310 © Springer Verlag 1980

Subject Index

List of Contributors

Buchhorn, Ing. (grad.) G.
Orthopädische Klinik, D-3400 Göttingen, Federal Republic of Germany

Ficat, Dr. P.
Chemin du Vallon, F-31000 Toulouse, France

Gérard, Prof. Y.
Clinique Chirurgicale Orthopédique et Traumatologique, F-51092 Reims Cedex,
France

Hori, Dr. Y.
Nara Medical University, Kashihara, Nara, Japan 634

Hungerford, Dr. D.S.
Johns Hopkins University, Maryland 21239, USA

Kotz, Doz. Dr. R.
Orthopädische Universitätsklinik, A-1090 Wien, Austria

Wagenhäuser, Prof. F.
Universitäts-Rheumaklinik Zürich, CH-8091 Zürich, Switzerland

Wagner, Prof. Dr. H.
Orthopädische Klinik Wichernhaus, Krankenhaus Rummelsberg,
D-8501 Schwarzenbruck, Federal Republic of Germany

Willert, Prof. Dr. H.-G.
Orthopädische Klinik, D-3400 Göttingen, Federal Republic of Germany

Zeiler, Dr. G.
Orthopädische Klinik Wichernhaus, Krankenhaus Rummelsberg,
D-8501 Schwarzenbruck, Federal Republic of Germany

Zichner, PD Dr. L.
Orthopädische Universitätsklinik Friedrichsheim, D-6000 Frankfurt a.M., Federal
Republic of Germany

Progress in Orthopaedic Surgery

Editorial Board: N. Gschwend, D. Hohmann,
J. L. Hughes, D. S. Hungerford, G. D. MacEwen,
E. Morscher, J. Schatzker, H. Wagner, U. H. Weil

Volume 1

Leg Length Discrepancy The Injured Knee

D. S. Hungerford
With contributions by numerous experts
1977. 100 figures. X, 160 pages
ISBN 3-540-08037-6

Contents: Leg Length Discrepancy: Basic Rehabilitation Principles of Persons with Leg Length Discrepancy: An Overview. Etiology and Pathophysiology of Leg Length Discrepancies. Measurement of Leg Length. Methodological Errors in Documenting Leg Length and Leg Length Discrepancies. Equalization of Leg Length with Orthopaedic Shoe Measures. Subtrochanteric Shortening and Lengthening Osteotomy. Surgical Lengthening or Shortening of Femur and Tibia. Technique and Indications. – The Injured Knee: The Importance of Arthrography Following Trauma to the Knee Joint. The Knee Joint of the Soccer Player (Its Stresses and Damages). Trauma-Induced Chondromalacia Patellae. Traumatic Injuries to the Articular Cartilage of the Knee.

Volume 2

Acetabular Dysplasia – Skeletal Dysplasias in Childhood

Editor: U. H. Weil
With contributions by numerous experts
1978. 133 figures, 20 tables. IX, 200 pages
ISBN 3-540-08400-2

Contents: Acetabular Dysplasia: Pathologic Anatomy of Congenital Hip Disease. Development and Clinical Importance of the Dysplastic Acetabulum. Radiologic Interpretation of Dysplasia of the Acetabulum. Femoral Osteotomies for Congenital Hip Dislocation. Our Experience with Salter's Innominate Osteotomy in the Treatment of Hip Dysplasia. Chiari Pelvic Osteotomy for Hip Dysplasia in Patients Below the Age of 20. Experiences with Spherical Acetabular Osteotomy for the Correction of the Dysplastic Acetabulum. Comparison of Pelvic Osteotomies in the Treatment of Congenital Hip Dislocation. – Skeletal Dysplasias in Childhood: Constitutional Disorders of Skeletal Development: The Skeletal Dysplasias Orthopaedic Corrections in Patients with Vitamin D-Resistant Rickets.

Volume 3

The Knee: Ligament and Articular Cartilage Injuries

Guesteditors: D. E. Hastings
With contributions by numerous experts
1978. 139 figures, 20 tables. X, 191 pages
ISBN 3-540-08679-X

Contents: Biomechanics and Pathophysiology. – The Acute Knee Ligament Injury. – Chronic Knee Ligament Instability. – The Acute Cartilage Injury. – The Old Cartilage Injury. – Retropatellar Cartilage Degeneration.

Volume 4

Joint Preserving Procedures of the Lower Extremity

Editor: U. H. Weil
With contributions by numerous experts.
1980. 87 figures, 9 tables. VIII, 121 pages
ISBN 3-540-09856-9

Contents: Resurfacing of the Hip Joint. – Long Term Results of Chiari Pelvic Osteotomies. – Results of Intertrochanteric Osteotomies in Patients with Coxarthrosis 12–15 Years After Surgery. – Long Term Results of Acetabular Shelf Arthroplasty. – Treatment of Osteoarthritis of the Knee by Osteotomy. – Principles of Corrective Osteotomies in Osteoarthrosis of the Knee. – Gait Analysis and its Benefit to the Patient. – Conservative Orthopaedic Management of Children with Myelomeningoceles. – Subject Index. – List of Contributors.

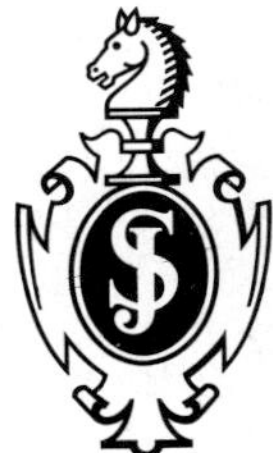

Springer-Verlag
Berlin
Heidelberg
New York

F. Séquin, R. Texhammar

AO/ASIF Instrumentation
Manual of Use and Care

Introduction and Scientific Aspects by H. Willenegger
Translated from the German by T. Telger

1981. Approx. 1300 figures, 17 separate Checklists.
XVI, 306 pages
ISBN 3-540-10337-6

Contents: Introduction. – Medical and Scientific Directives. – Principles of the AO (ASIF)-Technique and Basic Mechanical Principles. – Practical Part: Instrumentation of the AO/ASIF. Compressed Air and Compressed-Air Machines. Cleaning, Care, and Sterilization of Instruments and Implants. Preoperative, Operative, and Postoperative Guidelines. Suggestions for the Management of Various Fractures. – Preparation of the Instruments. – Subject Index.

The need for a practical guide to the use of AO instruments written with surgical assistants in mind has existed as long as the instruments themselves. This need is now met in *AO/ASIF Instrumentation.* It acquaints all members of the operating team with the goals and principles of AO/ASIF techniques while providing them with a comprehensive introduction to AO/ASIF instruments, their use and their maintenance. The book is arranged according to topic for easy reference, with carefully chosen illustrations rounding out the information in each section. Looseleaf tables are provided as checklists for laying out AO/ASIF instruments in the operating room. *AO/ASIF Instrumentation* supplements two other volumes in the Springer-Verlag program – *Manual of Internal Fixation and Small Fragment Set Manual –* and contains
- explanations of the scientific and clinical significance of AO/ASIF techniques
- detailed descriptions of individual implants and instruments
- instructions for the handling and use of implants and instruments
- directions for the care and maintenance of AO/ASIF instruments

This book will prove to be an indispensable reference for all surgical personnel concerned about the success fo internal fixation and the avoidance of methodologically induced failures.

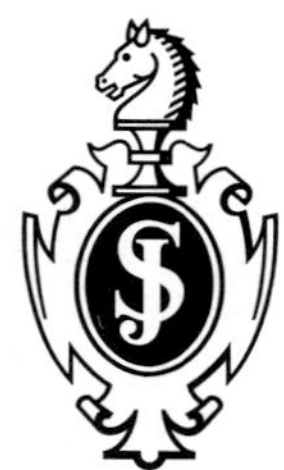

Springer-Verlag
Berlin
Heidelberg
New York